Pharmacy Registration
Assessment Questions 3

Pharmacy Registration Assessment Questions 3

Nadia Bukhari (Series Managing Editor)

BPharm, FRPharmS, FHEA, PG Dip Pharm Prac, PG Dip T&L in Higher Ed
Principal Teaching Fellow, UCL School of Pharmacy

Akila Ahmed (Contributor)

MPharmS, MSc Advanced Pharmacy Practice, IPres, Cert Advance
Clinical Practice
Lead Clinical Pharmacist for Women's and Child Health, Sandwell and
West Birmingham Hospitals NHS Trust

Dr Ryan Hamilton (Contributor)

MPharm (Hons), PGDip (Clinical Pharmacy), PGCert (Independent
Prescribing), PhD, MRPharmS, MFRPSI, AMRSC, AFHEA
Advanced Specialist Pharmacist in Antimicrobials, University Hospitals of
Leicester NHS Trust
Honorary Lecturer, School of Pharmacy, De Montfort University, Leicester

Sonia Kauser (Contributor)

PGCert (Advanced Clinical Practitioner), Independent Prescriber, PGCert
(Hospital Pharmacy), MPharm, Clinical Lecturer (University of
Manchester), Advanced Clinical Pharmacist Practitioner (Prescribing
Support Services)

Oksana Pyzik (Contributor)

MPharm, MRPharmS
Senior Teaching Fellow at the UCL School of Pharmacy in the Department
of Practice and Policy

Sadia Qayyum (Contributor)

BScPharmacy (Hons), PGCert (Clinical Pharmacy), MRPharmS, SFHEA,
Independent Prescriber, Lecturer in Pharmacy Practice (University of
Manchester), Relief Manager (Well Pharmacy), GP Practice Pharmacist,
Northern Lead for Primary Care Pharmacy Association

Pratik Thakkar (Contributor)

MPharm, MRPharmS
Medical Advisor - Oncology, Bristol-Myers Squibb

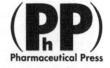

Pharmaceutical Press

Published by the Pharmaceutical Press
66–68 East Smithfield, London E1W 1AW, UK

© Pharmaceutical Press 2019

(**PP**) is a trade mark of Pharmaceutical Press

Pharmaceutical Press is the publishing division of the Royal Pharmaceutical
Society

First published 2019

Reprinted 2021

Typeset by Spi Global, Chennai, India
Printed in Great Britain by TJ Books Limited, Padstow, Cornwall

ISBN 978 0 85711 357 3 (print)
ISBN 978 0 85711 358 0 (mobi)
ISBN 978 0 85711 360 3 (epdf)
ISBN 978 0 85711 359 7 (ePub)

A catalogue record for this book is available from the British Library

---

Disclaimer
The views expressed in this book are solely those of the author
and do not necessarily reflect the views or policies of the Royal
Pharmaceutical Society. This book does NOT guarantee success
in the registration exam but can be used as an aid for revision.

To all the trainee pharmacists: stay true to yourselves, yet always open to learn.

Nadia Bukhari 2019

Contents

Preface

After the overwhelming success of our first four volumes of *Registration Exam Questions*, a decision was made to launch a new series named *Pharmacy Registration Assessment Questions* (PRAQ). In this new series we hope to incorporate questions that are aligned to the new GPhC Framework and incorporate a similar style of questions to what has recently been announced by the GPhC for the Registration Assessment.

Both editions of volume 1 have been well received, as well as volume 2, hence encouraging the writing of a new volume.

Volume 3 of PRAQ is a bank of just under 500 questions, which are similar to the style of the registration examination. The majority of the questions are based on law and ethics, and clinical pharmacy and therapeutic aspects of the registration examination syllabus, as well as pharmaceutical calculations.

After completing 4 years of study and graduating with a Master of Pharmacy (MPharm) degree, graduates are required to undertake training as a pre-registration pharmacist before they can sit the registration examination.

Pre-registration training is the period of employment on which graduates must embark and effectively complete before they can register as a pharmacist in the UK. In most cases it is a 1-year period after the pharmacy degree; for sandwich course students it is integrated within the undergraduate programme.

On successfully passing the registration examination, pharmacy graduates can register as a pharmacist in the UK.

The registration examination harmonises the testing of skills in practice during the pre-registration year. It tests:

- knowledge
- the application of knowledge
- calculation
- time management
- managing stress
- comprehension
- recall

- interpretation
- evaluation.

There are two examination papers: Paper 1 (calculations paper with extracts) and Paper 2 (closed book paper with extracts). Questions are based on practice-based situations and are designed to test the thinking and knowledge that lie behind any action.

EXAMINATION FORMAT

The registration examination consists of two papers:

1   Paper 1: calculations with extracts

- free text answers; calculators can be used (these are not provided by GPhC)
- 40 calculations in 120 minutes (2 hours)
- extracts from reference sources provided for questions that require additional information

2   Paper 2: closed book with extracts

- multiple-choice question (MCQ) paper with extracts from reference sources provided
- 120 questions in 150 minutes (2.5 hours)

Two types of MCQs are used:

- 90 single best answer questions
- 30 extended matching questions

The registration examination is crucial for pharmacy graduates wishing to register in the UK.

Due to student demand, *Pharmacy Registration Assessment Questions* will be an annual publication with brand-new questions for students to attempt. We hope to include questions on most aspects of the examination and will take any changes made by the GPhC into consideration.

Preparation is the key. This book cannot guarantee that you will pass the registration assessment; however, it can help you to identify your learning needs and practice questions with themes and elements from within the GPhC framework questions. And, as they say, 'practice makes perfect'.

This book is written with the most current *BNF* at the time of writing. Please use the most current *BNF* and reference sources when using this book.

Good luck with the preparation and the assessment.

Nadia Bukhari
January 2019

Acknowledgements

The editor wishes to acknowledge the support from colleagues at the UCL School of Pharmacy.

Thank you to all six contributors: Akila Ahmed, Ryan Hamilton, Sonia Kauser, Oksana Pyzik, Sadia Qayyum and Pratik Thakkar.

Nadia Bukhari would like to express thanks to the editors at Pharmaceutical Press for their support and patience in the writing of this book, and especially to Mark Pollard for his guidance.

About the authors

Nadia Bukhari BPharm, FRPharmS, FHEA, PG Dip Pharm Prac, PG Dip
T&L in Higher Ed

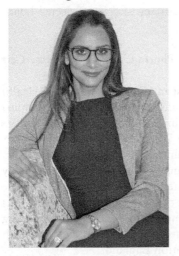

Nadia Bukhari is the Chair for the National RPS Pre-registration Conferences. She developed the extremely popular and over-subscribed conference when it first started in 2012. Nadia graduated from the School of Pharmacy, University of London, and after qualifying worked as a pharmacy manager at Westbury Chemist, Streatham for a year. She then moved on to work for Bart's and the London NHS Trust as a clinical pharmacist in surgery. It was at this time that Nadia developed an interest in teaching, because part of her role involved the responsibility of being a teacher practitioner for the School of Pharmacy, University of London. Two and a half years later, she commenced working for the School of Pharmacy, University of London as the pre-registration coordinator and the academic facilitator. This position involved teaching therapeutics to Master of Pharmacy students and assisting the director of undergraduate studies.

While teaching undergraduate students, Nadia completed her Post Graduate Diploma in Pharmacy Practice and her Post Graduate Diploma in Teaching in Higher Education. She then took on the role of the Master of Pharmacy Programme Manager, which involved the management of the undergraduate degree as well as being the pre-registration coordinator for the university.

Since the merger with UCL, Nadia is now a Principal Teaching Fellow in Pharmacy Practice and is the pre-registration coordinator and alumni coordinator for the university. She is also a Fellow of the Higher Education Academy and is the module lead for the final year pharmacy practice course.

Taking her research interest further, Nadia is currently in the fifth year of her PhD, which she is doing on a part-time basis. Her research area is 'leadership in pharmacy'.

Nadia's interest in writing emerged in her first year of working in academia. Thirteen years on, Nadia has authored eight titles with the Pharmaceutical Press. She is currently writing her ninth title, which is due to be published in March 2019.

Nadia is a Fellow of the Royal Pharmaceutical Society, in recognition of her distinction in the profession of pharmacy and is an elected board member for the English Pharmacy Board.

Akila Ahmed MPharmS, MSc Advanced Pharmacy Practice, IPres, Cert Advanced Clinical Practice
Akila Ahmed is a Lead Clinical Pharmacist in Women's and Child Health at Sandwell and West Birmingham Hospitals NHS Trust. She qualified in 2005 following a period of training in London at Imperial College Healthcare NHS Trust. She returned to the West Midlands to complete her junior training at Sandwell and West Birmingham Hospitals NHS Trust. During this time, Akila rotated through many clinical areas and quickly developed an interest in paediatrics, neonates and women's health. For the past six years she has worked on a number of strategic and clinical projects with medical colleagues in paediatrics, including education, developing guidelines within the acute sector across the West Midlands, working with CCGs, clinical networks and Health Education England.

In 2009, she took on a prescribing role at King's College London, where her initial scope of practice focused on immunology and infectious diseases. She has now expanded this further to provide expertise in clinical pharmaceutical care within women's and child health, and to support medical colleagues optimise the use of medicines across different care settings.

Within the West Midlands she has pioneered a number of innovative services for children and perinatal patients. Akila's other roles include pre-registration pharmacist tutor at Sandwell and West Birmingham Hospitals NHS Trust, member of the West Midlands Pre Registration Pharmacist Tutor Group, RPS Pre-registration Advisory Group member, Royal Pharmaceutical Society BNFC Quick Reference Guide lead author (published 2014) and National Hospital Pharmacy Programme panel member (CPPE England), developing and reviewing the national leadership and management programme for pharmacy professionals in England.

Dr Ryan Hamilton MPharm (Hons), PGDip (Clinical Pharmacy), PGCert (Independent Prescribing), PhD, MRPharmS, MFRPSI, AMRSC, AFHEA

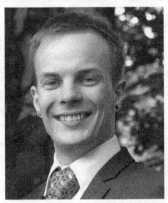

Ryan Hamilton is an Advanced Specialist Pharmacist in Antimicrobials & Acute Medicine at the University Hospitals of Leicester NHS Trust and an honorary lecturer at the School of Pharmacy, De Montfort University, Leicester.

Ryan studied pharmacy at Liverpool John Moore's University, to which he returned after completing his pre-registration training at King's College Hospital, London, to undertake a PhD in pharmaceutical sciences. His PhD research investigated the interaction of antimicrobial agents with clay minerals and the development of candidate materials for the treatment of infected wounds. Ryan's current research focuses on the optimal use of antimicrobial agents; from antimicrobial stewardship through to use in specialist populations. He also leads on antimicrobial resistance outreach projects locally and nationally; supporting the work of Antibiotic Research UK by sitting on the charity's education committee.

Throughout his career Ryan has supported pharmacy students and pre-registration pharmacists. As President of the British Pharmaceutical Students' Association, he developed guidance for students and trainees, and worked closely with the GPhC to ensure trainees were fairly represented. Ryan now acts as an ambassador for the BPSA and sits on the RPS's Faculty & Education Board where he continues to represent trainees and foundation year pharmacists.

Sonia Kauser MPharm, PG Dip Hosp Pharm, PG Dip (Advanced Clinical Practitioner, Independent Prescriber)

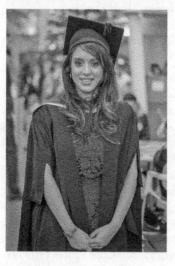

Sonia Kauser is currently a lecturer in Pharmacy Practice at the University of Manchester, a GP practice clinical pharmacist and an advanced clinical practitioner (minor ailments) at Prescribing Support Services.

She began her career as a pre-registration pharmacy student at Bradford Teaching Hospitals NHS Foundation Trust and then continued her role as a hospital pharmacist. She undertook training in various specialist rotations including paediatrics, oncology, psychiatry, general medicine, surgery, anticoagulation, cardiovascular and respiratory. She was able to pursue a postgraduate diploma in Clinical Hospital Pharmacy at the University of Bradford.

Sonia then transferred her skills to primary care in which she began the role of a clinical GP pharmacist (based in Yorkshire). This role enabled her to pursue Level 7 Independent Prescribing and her area of specialism was initially anticoagulation. This role has now developed and she undertakes various tasks including clinical medication reviews. She predominantly works as a clinical primary care pharmacist with an interest in anticoagulation and chronic disease management. She then decided to develop her skills and attained a postgraduate diploma in Advanced Practice – Clinical Practitioner, which allows her to manage minor ailment patients within a primary care or urgent care setting. This role allows her to work and support other healthcare professionals (such as GPs and nurses) by triaging patients and ensuring they are signposted to the correct services. This experience in primary care has allowed her to be part of national pilots for extended access/out of hours schemes.

Sonia has also worked in the following areas: urgent care, out of hours (walk-in centre), GSK (training of pharmaceutical reps), community pharmacy, acute ward pharmacist at Leeds Teaching Hospitals and guest lecturer role at the University of Bradford.

Sonia enjoys keeping active, reading and shopping in her spare time. Her most recent publication was in the *Prescriber Journal* June 2017 and describes the use of clinical information systems to improve practice within primary care.

Oksana Pyzik MPharm, MRPharmS

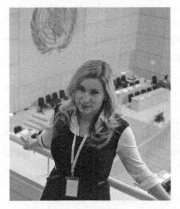

Oksana Pyzik is a Senior Teaching Fellow and Global Engagement Coordinator at University College London (UCL) School of Pharmacy. In addition to her role in education, Oksana is also a global health advisor and board trustee of the Commonwealth Pharmacists Association. Oksana first started her career as a pharmacist in the primary care setting delivering public health interventions to marginalised patient groups in underserved communities across London. It was this early experience in practice that motivated her to conduct public health research at the International Pharmaceutical Federation (FIP) before moving into the academic sector full time in 2013. She went on to earn her Post Graduate Diploma in Teaching and Learning in Higher Professional Education at the Institute of Education in 2015 and is now a Fellow of the UK Higher Education Academy. In 2017, Oksana was appointed as the FIP UCL FIPEd Collaborating Centre global engagement liaison in recognition of her leadership within pharmacy and global health. Oksana is extensively involved with the Royal Pharmaceutical Society (RPS) Pre-registration Conferences in both the development of teaching material and the delivery of training sessions. She also remains active in community pharmacy, serving as the pre-registration and academic lead for the Central London Local Practice Forum (LPF) where she acts as a link between community pharmacy and academia.

Sadia Qayyum BScPharmacy (Hons), PGCert (Clinical Pharmacy), MRPharmS, SFHEA, Independent Prescriber

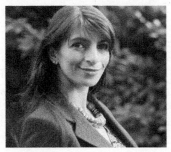

Sadia Qayyum has had extensive experience in retail, hospital and general practice in management and consultancy positions. She currently holds roles as lecturer in pharmacy practice at the University of Manchester, as an independent prescriber specialising in asthma for a number of general practices as well as a relief branch manager for Well. She is also the Northern lead for the Practice Pharmacists Group working with the Primary Care Pharmacists Association, as well being a committee member for the Kashmir Youth Project (KYP) in Rochdale.

From working in different disciplines of pharmacy along with other responsibilities held, she has experience of evaluating evidence and making objective decisions as well as good communication, intellectual and analytical skills. She displays commitment to equality, diversity and fair treatment by advising on and setting up policies and guidance in her various roles.

Speaking at career events to undergraduate pharmacy students, doctors and other professionals demonstrates Sadia's ability to learn, reflect and develop professionally. Often she is in a position to inspire the pharmacists of the future. Sadia has experience of coaching, mentoring and teaching a variety of healthcare professionals from diverse backgrounds and professions including pre-registration pharmacists, GP registrars, medical students, as well as other professionals through many of the roles held during her career.

Sadia continues to work to highlight the unique and invaluable role pharmacists have in healthcare. Irrespective of pharmacists sector of work, she wishes to champion the notion that all pharmacists should aspire to lead the profession into the future.

Pratik Thakkar MPharm, MRPharmS

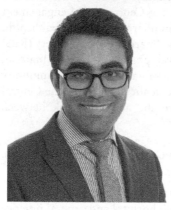

Pratik Thakkar graduated from UCL School of Pharmacy and completed his pre-registration placement at Great Ormond Street Hospital for Children.

After qualifying, he continued to work at Great Ormond Street as a Parenteral Nutrition and Quality Assurance Pharmacist. Following this, Pratik took an opportunity to work at the Medicines and Healthcare products Regulatory Agency (MHRA) in London in the Vigilance and Risk Management of Medicines department to gain further knowledge in pharmacovigilance (PV) and Regulatory Affairs.

He has also worked at Mylan Inc. in Product Safety and Risk Management. He was a PV pharmacist in the global pharmacovigilance function of the company, as well as in the medical affairs team. He worked on various projects to monitor the safety of the company's products on the market, as well as working on signing off material in line with the UK and Ireland Codes of Practice.

Pratik now works at Bristol-Myers Squibb where he has held various posts within Medical Governance and Compliance and Medical Affairs. He has gained experience in rheumatology and now oncology as a medical advisor. He has attained ABPI and IPHA final signatory status for UK and Irish business. He is actively involved in developing medical strategy for various oncology therapy indications and working closely with cross-functional teams and within the company to deliver innovative medicines for patients with serious and life-threatening diseases.

Abbreviations

ACBS	Advisory Committee on Borderline Substances
ACE	angiotensin-converting enzyme
ACEI	angiotensin-converting enzyme inhibitor
ACS	acute coronary syndrome
AF	atrial fibrillation
ALT DIE	alternate days
AV	arteriovenous
BD	twice daily
BMI	body mass index
BNF	*British National Formulary*
BNFC	*British National Formulary for Children*
BP	blood pressure
BPSA	British Pharmaceutical Students' Association
BSA	body surface area
BTS	British Thoracic Society
CCF	congestive/chronic cardiac failure
CD	controlled drug
CDC	US Centers for Disease Control and Prevention
CE	*conformité européenne*
CFC	chlorofluorocarbon
CHM	Commission on Human Medicines
CHMP	Committee for Medicinal Products for Human Use
CI	confidence interval or cumulative incidence
CKS	Clinical Knowledge Summaries
COX	cyclooxygenase
COPD	chronic obstructive pulmonary disease
CPD	continuing professional development
CPPE	Centre for Pharmacy Postgraduate Education
CrCl	creatinine clearance (mL/min)
CSM	Committee on Safety of Medicines
CYT	cytochrome
DigCl	digoxin clearance (L/h)
DMARD	disease-modifying antirheumatic drug
DNG	discount not given

DPF	*Dental Practitioners' Formulary*
DPI	dry-powder inhaler
EC	enteric-coated
ECG	electrocardiogram
EEA	European Economic Area
eGFR	estimated glomerular filtration rate
EHC	emergency hormonal contraception
F1	Foundation Year 1
FEV_1	forced expiratory volume in 1 second
GP	general practitioner
GP6D	glucose-6-phosphate dehydrogenase
GPhC	General Pharmaceutical Council
GSL	general sales list
GTN	glyceryl trinitrate
HbA1c	glycated haemoglobin
HDU	high dependency unit
HIV	human immunodeficiency virus
HR	heart rate
HRT	hormone replacement therapy
IBS	irritable bowel syndrome
IBW	ideal body weight
IDA	industrial denatured alcohol
IM	intramuscular
INR	international normalised ratio
IV	intravenous
IUD	intrauterine device
MAOI	monoamine oxidase inhibitor
MD	maximum single dose
MDD	maximum daily dose
MDI	metered-dose inhaler
MDU	to be used as directed
MEP	*Medicines, Ethics and Practice* guide
MHRA	Medicines and Healthcare products Regulatory Agency
MMR	measles, mumps and rubella
M/R	modified release
MRSA	meticillin-resistant *Staphylococcus aureus*
MUPS	multiple-unit pellet system
MUR	Medicines Use Review
NHS	National Health Service
NICE	National Institute for Health and Care Excellence
NMS	New Medicines Service
NRLS	National Reporting and Learning System

NSAIDs	non-steroidal anti-inflammatory drugs
OC	oral contraceptive
OD	*omni die* (every day)
OM	*omni mane* (every morning)
ON	*omni nocte* (every night)
OP	original pack
OPAT	outpatient parenteral antibacterial therapy
ORT	oral rehydration therapy
OTC	over-the-counter
P	pharmacy
PAGB	Proprietary Association of Great Britain
PCT	primary care trust
PHE	Public Health England
PIL	patient information leaflet
pMDI	pressurised metered-dose inhaler
PMR	patient medical record
POM	prescription-only medicine
POM-V	prescription-only medicine – veterinarian
POM-VPS	prescription-only medicine – veterinarian, pharmacist, suitably qualified person
PPIs	proton pump inhibitors
PRN	when required
PSA	prostate-specific antigen
PSNC	Pharmaceutical Services Negotiating Committee
QDS	*quarter die sumendum* (to be taken four times daily)
RCT	randomised controlled trial
RE	right eye
RPS	Royal Pharmaceutical Society (formerly RPSGB)
SARSS	Suspected Adverse Reaction Surveillance Scheme
SCRIPT	Standard Computerised Revalidation Instrument for Prescribing and Therapeutics
SeCr	serum creatinine
SGLT2	sodium (Na^+)/glucose co-transporter 2
SHO	senior house officer
SIGN	Scottish Intercollegiate Guidelines Network
SLS	selected list scheme
SOP	standard operating procedure
SPC	summary of product characteristics
SSRI	selective serotonin reuptake inhibitor
ST	an isoelectric line after the QRS complex of an ECG
STAT	immediately
TCA	tricyclic antidepressant

TDS	three times a day
TIA	transient ischaemic attack
TPN	total parenteral nutrition
TSDA	trade-specific denatured alcohol
U&E	urea and electrolyte count
UTI	urinary tract infection
VITAL	Virtual Interactive Teaching And Learning
WHO	World Health Organization

How to use this book

The book is divided into three main sections: single best answer questions, extended matching questions and calculation questions.

SINGLE BEST ANSWER QUESTIONS (SBAs)

Each of the questions or statements in this section is followed by five suggested answers. Select the best answer in each situation.

For example:
A patient on your ward has been admitted with a gastric ulcer, which is currently being treated. She has a history of arthritis and cardiac problems. Which of her drugs is most likely to have caused the gastric ulcer?

- ☐ A   paracetamol
- ☐ B   naproxen
- ☐ C   furosemide
- ☐ D   propranolol
- ☐ E   codeine phosphate

EXTENDED MATCHING QUESTIONS (EMQs)

Extended matching questions consist of lettered options followed by a list of numbered problems/questions. For each numbered problem/question, select the one lettered option that most closely answers the question. You can use the lettered options once, more than once or not at all.

For example:
Antidepressants

- A   amitriptyline
- B   citalopram
- C   duloxetine
- D   flupentixol

E   mirtazapine
F   moclobemide
G   St John's wort
H   venlafaxine

For questions 1–4
For the patients described, select the single most likely antidepressant from the list above. Each option may be used once, more than once or not at all.

1   Miss K is a 32-year-old woman on your ward who has a long-standing history of depression related to her chronic illness. She has tried antidepressants in the past but stopped them when she felt better. The medical team tell you that she returns to hospital periodically with relapsed symptoms because she stops taking her medicines. They want to treat her depression but the agent they suggest would not be suitable for Miss K, considering her non-adherence.

2   One of the new GPs in the surgery across the road calls you for some advice. He has a patient with him, Mr B, who is 28 years old and has agreed to try an antidepressant medicine. Mr B is otherwise fit and healthy, but the GP would like your advice on what to prescribe for this new diagnosis of moderate depression.

3   Three months later you get another call from the GP about Mr B, who has not responded well to the initial antidepressants and may be experiencing a number of side-effects. They want to switch him on to a different agent quickly, if not immediately. You inform the GP that one of the drugs he asked about cannot be started immediately.

4   Mrs C has just been admitted on to your emergency admissions unit after being referred directly from her GP, whom she went to see about her headache. On admission she also complains of palpitations and her BP is 205/100 mmHg. On taking her history you note she is Japanese and still eats a traditional diet, leading you to suspect her antidepressant medicine may have precipitated this condition.

CALCULATION QUESTIONS

These are free text pharmaceutical calculations. The use of calculators is permitted when tackling these questions. The GPhC will not provide candidates with calculators for the purpose of the assessment.

For example:

Mrs D is a 75-year-old woman who has just been admitted to your respiratory ward with an exacerbation of asthma. On admission she was weighed at 97 kg and states her height as 5 feet 3 inches. When taking her history you find she quit smoking 10 years ago and is on the following medicines:

Fostair 100/6 two puffs BD
Budesonide 4 mg PO OM
Phyllocontin Continus (aminophylline) 225-mg tablets, two tablets BD MDU
Salbutamol 2.5 mg nebulised QDS PRN
Salbutamol 100-mcg CFC-free inhaler 2–6 puffs QDS PRN via an aerochamber (blue)

How much aminophylline should Mrs D receive over the next 24 hours? Give your answer to the nearest whole number.

> The purpose of the registration assessment is to test a candidate's ability to apply the knowledge they have learnt over the past 5 years of their education and training.
>
> Testing someone's ability to locate information efficiently in the *BNF* should be tested during their pre-registration training year and in their undergraduate training.
>
> Therefore, all questions are closed book, with extracts of reference sources provided to candidates.

Answers to the questions are at the end of the book. Brief explanations or a suitable reference for sourcing the answer are given, to aid understanding and to facilitate learning.

Important: this text refers to the current edition of the *BNF* and *BNFC* when text was written. Please always consult the LATEST version for the most up-to-date information.

Single best answer questions

Akila Ahmed

1   A 76-year-old man is taking the following medicines:
   - simvastatin 40 mg once daily
   - atenolol 25 mg once daily
   - esomeprazole 40 mg once daily
   - metformin 500 mg twice daily
   - ramipril 2.5 mg once daily

   He has a history of type 2 diabetes, hypertension and IHD. He has just been diagnosed with severe peripheral vascular disease with symptoms of pain, achiness, fatigue, burning and discomfort in the muscles of the feet and calves.
   Which of his existing medicines would you consider to reduce and then eventually stop?

   - ☐ A   atorvastatin
   - ☐ B   atenolol
   - ☐ C   esomeprazole
   - ☐ D   metformin
   - ☐ E   ramipril

2   A 48-year-old Caucasian man has been diagnosed with hypertension. His BP is 160/100 mmHg. He is starting antihypertensive therapy. He does not have any other medical conditions and has no known allergies.
   What is the most appropriate first-line anti-hypertensive for this man?

   - ☐ A   amlodipine
   - ☐ B   bisoprolol

    ☐ C   doxazosin
    ☐ D   indapamide
    ☐ E   ramipril

3   A 4-year-old child with no long-term medical conditions requires paracetamol for the treatment of pyrexia associated with flu-like symptoms. What is the most appropriate dose of paracetamol to be administered every 6 hours?

    ☐ A   60 mg
    ☐ B   120 mg
    ☐ C   180 mg
    ☐ D   240 mg
    ☐ E   360 mg

4   A patient with type 1 diabetes has been on oral medication to manage his diabetes. However, because his HbA1c is very high the GP decides to change the therapy and decides to prescribe insulin. The doctor wants an insulin that is long acting and could be administered once a day. This patient has poor glucose control during the day and night and does not like injecting too often.

    Which of the following is the most suitable insulin preparation for this person?

    ☐ A   *Actrapid®* (soluble insulin)
    ☐ B   *Apidra®* (insulin glulisine)
    ☐ C   *Humalog Mix25®* (biphasic insulin lispro)
    ☐ D   *Lantus®* (insulin glargine)
    ☐ E   *NovoRapid®* (insulin aspart)

Questions 5–8 relate to Mr Robinson, a 91-year-old man who was admitted with an infected toe and was treated with a 7 day course of flucloxacillin 500 mg four times. Mr Robinson was found unresponsive by the nursing staff.

- Past medical history: type 2 diabetes, hypercholesterolemia, peripheral vascular disease
- Drug history: aspirin 75 mg once a day, gliclazide 80 mg twice a day, metformin 850 mg three times a day, simvastatin 40 mg once at night, co-codamol 30/500 1–2 four times a day when required
- Social history: non-smoker and drinks 30–40 units of alcohol per week
- NKDA

- Observation: temperature 38.1°C, HR 100 beats/min, BP 136/81 mmHg, RR 20 beats/min
- Blood glucose: 2.1 mmol/L (3.9–7.8)
- Sodium: 139 mmol/L (137–145)
- Serum potassium: 4.1 mmol/L (3.5–5.1)
- Serum urea: 6.2 mmol/L (2.5–7.5)
- Serum creatinine: 80 micromol/L (46–92)
- Estimated GFR: 90 mL/min/1.73 m^2 (>60)

5   Which of the following conditions below is this patient experiencing?

- □ A   hyperglycaemia
- □ B   hyperkalaemia
- □ C   hypernatraemia
- □ D   hyponatraemia
- □ E   hypoglycaemia

6   In Mr Robinson's case, which of the following is the most likely explanation that could be contributing to the patient's symptoms?

- □ A   Aspirin in conjunction with a change in his diet associated with the hospital admission
- □ B   Co-codamol in conjunction with a change in his diet associated with the hospital admission
- □ C   Gliclazide in conjunction with a change in his diet associated with the hospital admission
- □ D   Metformin in conjunction with a change in his diet associated with the hospital admission
- □ E   Simvastatin in conjunction with a change in his diet associated with the hospital admission

7   Which one of the following can be used to treat this patient's presenting symptoms?

- □ A   gliclazide
- □ B   glucagon
- □ C   glycogen
- □ D   insulin
- □ E   metformin

8   The doctor explains that Mr Robinson has patterns of hypoglycaemic attacks at a particular time and asks for your advice.

Which of the following recommendations would you suggest?

☐ A   Add a dose of insulin before the time of hypoglycaemia and monitor blood glucose regularly

☐ B   Add in alogliptin 25 mg once a day

☐ C   Change gliclazide to glipizide for administration before the time of hypoglycaemia and blood glucose monitored regularly

☐ D   Do nothing and just monitor the patient

☐ E   Increase the dose of gliclazide scheduled for administration before the time of hypoglycaemia and blood glucose monitored regularly

9   Mrs SJ is a 43-year-old woman who asks to speak to a pharmacist because she wants something for her stomach ache. You find out that the pain is located in the lower and upper left quadrant. She is on the following medication:

- paracetamol taken when required for 6 months for knee pain
- lactulose when required
- cetirizine for allergic rhinitis
- atorvastatin 20 mg at night for familial hyperlipidaemia
- naproxen 500 mg twice a day as needed; she has taken this for 2 weeks for knee pain as well

You reach a differential diagnosis of non-ulcer dyspepsia.
What medicine could potentially be causing these symptoms?

☐ A   paracetamol

☐ B   atorvastatin

☐ C   naproxen

☐ D   cetirizine

☐ E   lactulose

Questions 10 and 11 relate to a 35-year-old woman's pre-pregnancy state. Her weight is 80 kg and she has a CrCl of 84 mL/min in her third trimester of pregnancy. She has been found to have a pulmonary embolism. She has no life-threatening symptoms but needs to start on a low molecular weight heparin (LMWH).

10   Which of the following enoxaparin dose is correct?

☐ A   enoxaparin injection 40 mg SC once daily

☐ B   enoxaparin injection 80 mg SC once daily

☐ C   enoxaparin injection 120 mg SC once daily

     □ D   enoxaparin injection 75 mg SC twice daily
     □ E   enoxaparin injection 80 mg SC twice daily

11 Which one of the following side effects is caused by enoxaparin?

     □ A   dry mouth
     □ B   hyponatraemia
     □ C   jaundice
     □ D   nausea
     □ E   thrombocytopenia

Questions 12–14 relate to a 31-year-old man with increased seizures who was admitted 6 days ago with recurrent complex partial seizures.

- PMH: focal epilepsy
- DH: phenytoin 300 mg daily, Keppra 1.5 g BD
- No known allergies
- Non-smoker and no alcohol consumption

Phenytoin was started with an initial 1.5 grams intravenous loading dose and oral phenytoin 300 mg tablets as a maintenance dose thereafter. The neurology team advises to aim to achieve a serum phenytoin concentration in the upper half of the target range.

12 Which of the following is the normal target range for phenytoin?

     □ A   8–10 mg/L
     □ B   7–15 mg/L
     □ C   10–20 mg/L
     □ D   8–20 mg/L
     □ E   2–5 mg/L

Results for blood investigations were:

- creatinine – normal
- eGFR – normal
- albumin – 38 g/L (35–48)
- after 5 days of treatment the serum phenytoin was 12.9 microgram/mL (10–20)

The junior doctor wants some help with reviewing the phenytoin dosage in light of the drug concentration data and neurology advice.

13 Which of the following advice would be appropriate?

     □ A   Double the dose of phenytoin so the drug concentration doesn't decrease

□ **B**   Increase the dose of phenytoin from 300 mg to 350 mg
□ **C**   Increase the phenytoin dose frequency to twice a day
□ **D**   The dose of phenytoin should not be adjusted because the drug concentration is within the target range
□ **E**   Wait for another 5 days before you adjust the dose

14 The doctor wants to change the phenytoin tablet formulation to phenytoin liquid.
What dose should be prescribed?

□ **A**   300 mg
□ **B**   312 mg
□ **C**   322 mg
□ **D**   333 mg
□ **E**   350 mg

Questions 15–17 relate to Mrs Dennis, a 90-year-old woman who was admitted to hospital following a fall. She bruised her hip but had no fracture. She has a history of hypothyroidism, hypercholesterolemia, osteoarthritis and myocardial infarction.

- Drug history: clopidogrel 75 mg, levothyroxine 100 mcg once a day, atorvastatin 40 mg once a day, ramipril 5 mg once a day, naproxen 500 mg twice a day, temazepam 10 mg at night and paracetamol 1 grams four times a day when required
- NKDA
- On observation BP lying 124/68 and standing 98/56 mmHg

15 In light of her fall, which one of the following drugs would you change?

□ **A**   atorvastatin
□ **B**   clopidogrel
□ **C**   levothyroxine
□ **D**   paracetamol
□ **E**   ramipril

16 Due to the fall and previous history of osteoarthritis the medical team decide to continue the use of naproxen for pain relief.
Select the most likely possible consequence from the list if they continue to prescribe naproxen.

□ **A**   bleeding risk increased
□ **B**   bradycardia
□ **C**   constipation

□ D diarrhoea
□ E hypertensive crisis

Mrs Dennis's blood investigation results were made available:

- Sodium: 136 mmol/L (135–145)
- Potassium: 4.7 mmol/L (3.5–4.7)
- Creatinine: 118 micromol/L (60–110)
- e-GFR: 40 mL/min/1.73 m^2

17 In light of the blood investigations, which medication needs to be reviewed?

□ A atorvastatin
□ B clopidogeral
□ C levothyroxine
□ D naproxen
□ E paracetamol

Questions 18–19 relate to Mr JG, a 60-year-old male who has been complaining of a swollen red toe that has become increasingly swollen over the last 24 hours. Two weeks ago he was started on a new hypertensive drug to achieve a better blood pressure. His past medical history includes hypertension, osteoarthritis, gout and heart failure. His medication includes allopurinol 100 mg OD, bisoprolol 5 mg OD, isosorbide mononitrate XL 60 mg OD, bendroflumethiazide 2.5 mg OD, ramipril 10 mg OD and co-codamol 30/500 2 QDS. A diagnosis of gout is made.

18 Which of the following medications should be prescribed for Mr JG to address his inflamed toe?

□ A allopurinol
□ B aspirin
□ C colchicine
□ D naproxen
□ E paracetamol

19 Which of the following drugs do you think may have precipitated the symptoms?

□ A allopurinol
□ B bendroflumethiazide
□ C bisoprolol
□ D isosorbide mononitrate XL
□ E ramipril

20 A 60 kg patient with endocarditis receives intravenous gentamicin at 5 mg/kg in three divided doses (100 mg 8 hourly). Two doses have been administered (target for gentamicin: trough <1 mg/L). Gentamicin trough concentration was 1.8 mg/L.

Which of the following is an appropriate method of dose rationalisation?

    □ A   Decrease the dose and decrease the dosage interval
    □ B   Increase the dose and increase the dosage interval
    □ C   Increase the dose and maintain the same dosage interval
    □ D   Maintain the same dose and increase the dosage interval
    □ E   Maintain the same dose and decrease the dosage interval

21 A 65-year-old man who has COPD and persistent breathlessness is now finding it difficult to walk to the local shops. He is a lifelong smoker and currently smokes 25 cigarettes a day. He was using an ipratropium metered dose inhaler (20 micrograms/metered inhalation) as required, but this is being discontinued by his GP since it no longer controls his symptoms. His FEV_1 is greater than 50% predicted.
Which of the following is the most appropriate treatment?
You may use NICE guidance on chronic obstructive pulmonary disease in over 16s: diagnosis and management (NG115) to help you.

    □ A   *Clenil Modulite*® metered dose inhaler (beclometasone dipropionate 100 micrograms)
    □ B   fluticasone propionate metered dose inhaler (250 micrograms)
    □ C   salbutamol metered dose inhaler (100 micrograms)
    □ D   *Seretide*® 250 Accuhaler (fluticasone propionate 250 micrograms and salmeterol xinafoate)
    □ E   *Spiriva Respimat*® 2.5 micrograms/dose solution for inhalation cartridge with device

22 A 2-year-old with a peanut allergy who weighs 18 kg was seen in the outpatient clinic and experiences anaphylaxis, which is an emergency. What dose of intramuscular adrenaline auto injector would you prescribe for this child for use in an emergency?

    □ A   Administer adrenaline 100 micrograms
    □ B   Administer adrenaline 150 micrograms
    □ C   Administer adrenaline 250 micrograms
    □ D   Administer adrenaline 300 micrograms
    □ E   Administer adrenaline 500 micrograms

Questions 23–25 relate to a 78-year-old man with COPD and ischaemic heart disease. He is admitted to hospital from home with shortness of breath and over the last 3 days he has had a bad cough. His sputum has changed colour from grey to dark green. He has become progressively more short of breath. He began taking antibiotics the day before admission. His blood pressure on admission is 128/58 mmHg. He has no known drug allergies and his current medication is listed on his hospital inpatient prescription chart: *Relvar Ellipta*® (fluticasone furoate 184 micrograms/vilanterol 22 micrograms inhalation powder) 1 puff inhaled daily, isosorbide mononitrate M/R 60 mg oral daily, ramipril 10 mg oral daily, aspirin 75 mg oral daily, *Clexane*® (enoxaparin sodium) 40 mg SC daily, salbutamol 100 micrograms/inhalation 2 puffs inhaled PRN.

23 Microbiology results are not yet available but an atypical pathogen is not suspected.
    What is the most likely cause of this man's respiratory tract infection?

    ☐ A *Chlamydia psittaci*
    ☐ B *Legionella pneumophilia*
    ☐ C *Mycoplasma pneumoniae*
    ☐ D *Pneumocystis jirovecii*
    ☐ E *Streptococcus pneumoniae*

24 During his admission, he complains that for several weeks now he has had a sore mouth.
    Which of the following drugs is the most likely cause of his sore mouth?

    ☐ A aspirin
    ☐ B isosorbide mononitrate
    ☐ C ramipril
    ☐ D *Relvar Ellipta*®
    ☐ E salbutamol

25 Which oral antibiotic is most likely to be prescribed for this patient with an exacerbation of COPD?

    ☐ A doxycycline
    ☐ B fucidic acid
    ☐ C metronidazole
    ☐ D phenoxymethylpenicillin
    ☐ E vancomycin

26 A 48-year-old man was admitted with dizziness and feeling faint. His past medical history includes depression, psychosis, diet-controlled diabetes and allergic rhinitis. His medication includes paracetamol 1 g QDS, docusate, codeine 30 mg QDS, cetrizine 10 mg OD, olanzapine 20 mg OD, mometasone spray. On admission his ECG showed an abnormal rhythm with QT prolongation.
Which of the following could be the cause of the presenting symptoms?

    ☐ A   cetirizine
    ☐ B   docusate
    ☐ C   mometasone
    ☐ D   olanzipine
    ☐ E   paracetamol

27 A 32-year-old female who has pre-existing hypertension and is 20 weeks pregnant.
Which of the following medicines would be the most appropriate to manage her blood pressure which is 160/100 mmHg?

    ☐ A   atenolol
    ☐ B   carvedilol
    ☐ C   labetalol
    ☐ D   losartan
    ☐ E   ramipril

Questions 28 and 29 relate to a 29-year-old woman who is in pain following an operation. She has no past medical history and is not on any medication before admission. Following the surgery she was on maximum doses of analgesia; ibuprofen 400 mg TDS, paracetamol 1 gram QDS and *Oramorph*® 2.5 mg every 2 hours regularly. However, despite the analgesics she is still experiencing severe pain (defined 7/10). The local analgesics guidelines include the WHO pain ladder to manage patients.

28 She prefers to take oral medication. Which of the following options would be the most appropriate intervention to manage her pain?

    ☐ A   Add in a weak opioid like codeine
    ☐ B   Increase the dose of ibuprofen to QDS
    ☐ C   Increase the *Oramorph*® 5 mg 2 hourly PRN
    ☐ D   Make no changes and the pain will get better
    ☐ E   Prescribe and add in a regular sustained release i.e. morphine sulphate

29 What dose of regular sustained release morphine sulphate (*MST Continus®*) should be prescribed in addition to the existing analgesics?

    □ **A**   *MST Continus®* 5 mg 12 hourly
    □ **B**   *MST Continus®* 7.5 mg 12 hourly
    □ **C**   *MST Continus®* 10 mg 12 hourly
    □ **D**   *MST Continus®* 15 mg 12 hourly
    □ **E**   *MST Continus®* 20 mg 12 hourly

30 A 2 kg baby requires dobutamine at a dose of 10 micrograms/kg/min. The rate at which the infusion will run is 0.2 mL/hr. The final volume of the syringe is 50 mL (dobutamine + glucose 5%).
How many millilitres of dobutamine 12.5 mg/mL are needed for this infusion?

    □ **A**   2.4 mL
    □ **B**   24 mL
    □ **C**   30 mL
    □ **D**   240 mL
    □ **E**   300 mL

31 You are a pharmacist on call and the neonatal nurse requests a fluid bag for a neonate with low potassium. The bag requested contains potassium chloride 10 mmol in sodium chloride 0.9% and glucose 5%. You realise there is no stock of a ready-made bag and will need to advise the nurse on how to prepare the bag. You need potassium chloride 10 mmol in sodium chloride 0.9% and glucose 5% 500 mL (Bag A). You have a bag containing potassium chloride 10 mmol in glucose 5% available (Bag B).
How much 30% sodium chloride (5 mmol/mL) would you add to bag B to make up the requested fluid for bag A?

    □ **A**   12.5 mL
    □ **B**   15.0 mL
    □ **C**   16.4 mL
    □ **D**   17.5 mL
    □ **E**   20.5 mL

Questions 32 and 33 relate to Mr MM who is looking after his 8-year-old grandson for the weekend. He attends his local pharmacy and wants some advice; he noticed a rash this morning when he was dressing him. During the pharmacy consultation you identify the rash on his face and that it has spread across his back in clusters of small red lumps and some fluid-filled vesicles, but no blisters. The 8-year-old said he finds the rash extremely itchy, feels tired and has a fever.

32 What do you think is the likely diagnosis?

    ☐ A   chicken pox
    ☐ B   dermatitis
    ☐ C   impetigo
    ☐ D   measles
    ☐ E   mumps

33 Which organism causes the rash?

    ☐ A   Epstein-Barr virus
    ☐ B   herpes simplex virus
    ☐ C   herpes varicella zoster
    ☐ D   molluscum contagiosum
    ☐ E   *Staphylococcus aureus*

Questions 34–36 relate to a 15-month-old girl weighing 12 kg with gastroenteritis who was admitted yesterday with vomiting and diarrhoea. The child has been assessed by the paediatric registrar who estimates that the child is 5% dehydrated. The registrar's documents contain notes for the junior team to prescribe intravenous fluids to cover maintenance requirements and to correct the child's fluid deficit over the 24 hours.

You may use the BNFC monograph for fluids and electrolytes to help you: https://www.formularycomplete.com/view/treatmentsummary/monograph/118868

34 What is the maintenance fluid requirement for this child?

    ☐ A   110 mL/day
    ☐ B   1000 mL/day
    ☐ C   1100 mL/day
    ☐ D   1900 mL/day
    ☐ E   2000 mL/day

35 You also need to replace the existing deficit. The child is estimated to be 5% dehydrated. What is the deficit?

    ☐ A   50 mL
    ☐ B   72 mL
    ☐ C   120 mL
    ☐ D   500 mL
    ☐ E   600 mL

36 What is the daily fluid requirement for this child? Daily fluid requirement (mL) = maintenance + deficit.

    □ A   500 mL
    □ B   600 mL
    □ C   1100 mL
    □ D   1650 mL
    □ E   1700 mL

37 Which of the following is a toxoid vaccine?

    □ A   diphtheria
    □ B   hepatitis B
    □ C   Hib (haemophilus influenzae type b) disease
    □ D   HPV (human papillomavirus)
    □ E   pneumococcal disease

Questions 38–39 relate to a 46-year-old Afro-Caribbean man who works as a bus driver visited his GP following concerns about his blood pressure. He had three separate high blood pressure readings, has a strong family history of cardiovascular risk and was diagnosed with hypertension.

38 Which of the following medicines would be the most appropriate?

    □ A   amlodipine
    □ B   atenolol
    □ C   doxazocin
    □ D   furosemide
    □ E   ramipril

39 Which of the following is the most common long-term side effect that the patient should be counselled about?

    □ A   alopecia
    □ B   anaemia
    □ C   ankle swelling
    □ D   sore mouth
    □ E   vomiting and diarrhoea

40 Marie is an 84-year-old woman with hypertension and rheumatoid arthritis. She lives at home on her own. She also receives daily support from a care worker to help with activities of daily living. She is currently prescribed:

- bendroflumethiazide 2.5 mg daily
- simvastatin 20 mg at night

- methotrexate 20 mg once weekly on a Wednesday
- folic acid 5 mg daily except on Wednesday
- paracetamol 1 four times a day when required

She receives a home visit from the GP who diagnoses a urinary tract infection (UTI) and prescribes trimethoprim 200 mg twice daily for 3 days. On Sunday, the care worker is very concerned that Marie has deteriorated and is feeling very sick and confused with delirium. Marie has developed acute renal injury and pancytopenia.

Which of the following drugs caused Marie's condition to deteriorate?

- ☐ A   bendroflumethiazide
- ☐ B   folic acid
- ☐ C   paracetamol
- ☐ D   simvastatin
- ☐ E   trimethoprim

SECTION B

Ryan Hamilton

1   Mrs G has just been transferred to a side-room after suffering two episodes of diarrhoea, which the medical team are suspecting to be *Clostridium difficile* infection.
   Which of her medicines should you advise the medical team to withhold?

    ☐ A   bisoprolol
    ☐ B   candesartan
    ☐ C   omeprazole
    ☐ D   simvastatin
    ☐ E   zopiclone

2   Miss J has been admitted to your acute medical unit with confusion. You complete her drug history and find she is taking sodium valproate and citalopram. When checking her bloods you find one of her biochemical markers is out of range, contributing to her confusion.
   Which of the following is most likely to be causing her confusion?
   You may use the SPC for *Epilim*® 200 mg tablets to help you: http://www.medicines.org.uk/emc/medicine/23021

    ☐ A   hypoglycaemia
    ☐ B   hypokalaemia
    ☐ C   hyponatraemia
    ☐ D   hypophosphataemia
    ☐ E   none of the above

3   You are a pharmacist working in a GP surgery when one of the general practitioners comes in to talk to you about one of his diabetic patients. This patient has recently been discharged from hospital after suffering from diabetic ketoacidosis. However, her blood glucose levels have been well controlled and were not raised during the DKA and the GP asks for your insight.
   Which of the patient's medicines is likely to have precipitated the DKA?

    ☐ A   aspirin
    ☐ B   dapagliflozin
    ☐ C   gliclazide
    ☐ D   metformin
    ☐ E   ramipril

4 Mr O has been diagnosed with cancer to be treated with vincristine and one of the junior doctors asks for your advice on how to administer this medicine.
Which of the following routes must vincristine be administered by?

☐ A   intrathecal
☐ B   intravenous
☐ C   oral
☐ D   rectal
☐ E   subcutaneous

5 Ms Y presents to your community pharmacy with a new prescription for methotrexate 10 mg weekly and folic acid 5 mg weekly. She asks you how to take these tablets.
Which of the following would you NOT tell her?
You may use the folic acid monograph in the BNF to help you answer this question.

☐ A   Take the folic acid on the same day as the methotrexate
☐ B   Take the folic acid the day after the methotrexate
☐ C   Take the folic acid the day before the methotrexate
☐ D   Take the folic acid 2 days after the methotrexate
☐ E   Take the folic acid 3 days after the methotrexate

Questions 6–8 concern Miss J who is being treated for depression and has not responded to amitriptyline.

6 Miss J does not want to take citalopram because it did not help her friend so her GP has prescribed phenelzine instead. You find that Miss J has not been counselled on how to take this new medicine and you decide to contact her GP.
Which of the following would be the most important to discuss with the GP?

☐ A   Which brand of phenelzine to supply
☐ B   Which day the amitriptyline should stop and the phenelzine commence
☐ C   Which day the patient is due back for a review
☐ D   Which food and drink the patient should avoid
☐ E   Which side effects the patient should be counselled on

7 When handing the phenelzine over to Miss J you decide to counsel her on what dietary considerations she needs to make. You enquire about her diet and what food, drink and treats she enjoys.

Which of the following food is Miss J safe to ingest while taking moclobemide?

    ☐ A   blue cheese
    ☐ B   olives
    ☐ C   salami
    ☐ D   soya beans
    ☐ E   tofu

8   Three months later, Miss J is taken to hospital by ambulance after falling unwell. On admission she was described as becoming quickly agitated and aggressive and was suffering from involuntary muscle spasms and hyperthermia. When speaking to her partner you find that Miss J had taken one of her partner's venlafaxine tablets by mistake. Which of the following conditions is Miss J likely suffering from?

    ☐ A   hypertensive crisis
    ☐ B   Korsakoff's psychosis
    ☐ C   neuroleptic malignant syndrome
    ☐ D   sepsis
    ☐ E   serotonin syndrome

9   Mrs L comes into your pharmacy with a new prescription for amiodarone.
Which of the following is the most important piece of advice to give Mrs L?
You may use the SPC for amiodarone 100 mg tablets to help you: https://www.medicines.org.uk/emc/product/6019

    ☐ A   All of the below
    ☐ B   Avoid high potassium containing foods
    ☐ C   Do not drive at night as she may get dazzled by headlights
    ☐ D   Tablets can be crushed and taken with yoghurt
    ☐ E   Wear sun cream, even on a cloudy day

10   Mr P is a 43-year-old man of African descent who takes metformin 1 g BD for non-insulin dependent diabetes mellitus. His blood pressure has been persistently above 140 mmHg systolic and greater than 90 mmHg diastolic, and his GP would like to start antihypertensive treatment. Which of the following would be the initial treatment of choice?

    ☐ A   amlodipine 5 mg OD
    ☐ B   amlodipine 5 mg OD and candesartan 8 mg OD
    ☐ C   amlodipine 5 mg OD and ramipril 2.5 mg OD
    ☐ D   candesartan 8 mg OD
    ☐ E   ramipril 2.5 mg OD

11 Mrs N is a 63-year-old woman who continues to smoke ten cigarettes per day after numerous failed attempts to stop smoking. Over the past five years she has managed her COPD with a salbutamol CFC free inhaler, which she uses when required for breathlessness. However, her breathing has gotten worse and her FEV_1 has come back as 64% of predicted.
Which agent should be added onto her treatment?

☐ A   *QVAR®* (beclometasone) 100 mcg/dose pMDI, one dose BD

☐ B   *Seretide®* (fluticasone and salmeterol) 500 Accuhaler, one dose BD

☐ C   *Spiriva®* (tiotropium) 18 mcg/dose DPI, one dose OD

☐ D   *Symbicort®* (budesonide and formoterol) 400/12 Turbohaler, one dose BD

☐ E   *Trimbow®* (beclometasone, formoterol, and glycopyrronium) 87/5/9 pMDI 2 doses BD

12 You are working in a community pharmacy when a member of the public rushes in for help as her friend has collapsed. You attend the scene and find a 57-year-old woman unconscious on the floor. After determining that she is unconscious and instructing the woman to dial 999 you begin CPR.
What ratio of rescue breaths to chest compressions should you perform?

☐ A   1 breath per 10 compressions

☐ B   1 breath per 20 compressions

☐ C   1 breath per 30 compressions

☐ D   2 breaths per 20 compressions

☐ E   2 breaths per 30 compressions

13 Mrs H comes into your community pharmacy with a prescription for ileostomy bags. Her stoma was formed from the upper part of her ileum during an emergency hospital admission 4 weeks ago. Whilst waiting for the items to be dispensed you talk to Mrs H about how she is coping with her new ileostomy and she complains that her stoma became partially blocked over the weekend.
Which of the following foods is more likely to cause blockages in stomas?

☐ A   broccoli

☐ B   cabbage

☐ C   cucumber

☐ D   potato

☐ E   tomato

14 Mr H is a patient on your ward who has been admitted with a blood glucose level of 11.7 mmol/L.
Which of his medicines is most likely to cause the fluctuation in blood glucose levels?

  □ A   aspirin
  □ B   bendroflumethiazide
  □ C   paracetamol
  □ D   ramipril
  □ E   tramadol

15 Miss L comes to your pharmacy complaining of nausea. On questioning, she tells you that she is around 5 weeks pregnant.
Which of the following would be the most appropriate course of action?

  □ A   None of the below
  □ B   Supply cyclizine
  □ C   Supply *Gaviscon Advance*®
  □ D   Supply prochlorperazine
  □ E   Supply promethazine

16 Mrs S comes into your pharmacy complaining of a sore throat, which she has had for 3 days. While interviewing her about her sore throat you find out that she has had some *Tunes*, which only gave temporary relief. She would like you to suggest an over-the-counter remedy for her. You ask her if she is on any other medication and she tells you that she takes carbimazole 5 mg daily and propranolol 10 mg three times daily for hyperthyroidism.
Which of the following is the most appropriate advice for this patient?

  □ A   Drink plenty of water as OTC products have insufficient clinical evidence
  □ B   Gargle with dispersible aspirin
  □ C   Refer Mrs S to her GP
  □ D   Take paracetamol
  □ E   Take simple linctus

17 You have recently started working with another pharmacist but have some serious concerns about their behaviour and performance. You believe that patient care may be put at risk.
Which of the following should you NOT do when initially raising your concerns?

  □ A   Keep a record
  □ B   Maintain confidentiality

☐ C   Report to the GPhC
☐ D   Report to the other pharmacist's supervisor
☐ E   Report to your supervisor

18 Mrs S gives you a veterinary prescription. It is for *Otomax*® (gentamicin compound) ear drops for her pet dog Rover, who has an ear infection. You find out that *Otomax*® is licensed for the treatment of acute external otitis in dogs.
Which of the following particulars does NOT legally need to be written on the prescription?

☐ A   Qualification of the prescriber
☐ B   Name/identification of the animal to be treated
☐ C   Species of the animal to be treated
☐ D   Name and address of the animal's owner
☐ E   Statement that the drug was prescribed under the veterinary cascade

19 Mrs Y comes to your pharmacy one afternoon asking for some advice. Her 7-year-old daughter has had two small episodes of diarrhoea that morning and would like something to treat it. Her daughter is otherwise well and there are no immediate warning signs.
What is the most appropriate course of action?

☐ A   Advise on increased fluid intake
☐ B   Refer to GP
☐ C   Supply loperamide
☐ D   Supply oral rehydration sachets
☐ E   Supply *Pepto-Bismol*®

20 Mr D has been diagnosed with cellulitis and requires oral antibacterial therapy to treat it. The senior house officer asks for your advice on the ward round with regards to choice of the antibacterial. You check the patient's notes and find out that the patient has a history of anaphylaxis with penicillin.
Which of the following drugs would be most suitable?

☐ A   cefalexin
☐ B   clarithromycin
☐ C   co-amoxiclav
☐ D   flucloxacillin
☐ E   meropenem

21 Mr H has been newly prescribed atorvastatin 10 mg tablets. The GP's instruction is to 'take one tablet once a day'. Mr H asks you when he should take the tablet.
What should you advise?

    ☐ **A**　Any of the below
    ☐ **B**　None of the below
    ☐ **C**　Take in the afternoon
    ☐ **D**　Take in the evening
    ☐ **E**　Take in the morning

22 You are working on an orthopaedic ward and one of your patients, Mrs Q, is about to be prescribed daptomycin IV at a dose of 6 mg/kg daily. You know that this medicine requires close monitoring to prevent harm and adverse effects.
Which of the following serum parameters must be measured before and throughout treatment?
You may use the SPC for daptomycin to help you: https://www .medicines.org.uk/emc/product/8124/smpc

    ☐ **A**　blood urea nitrogen
    ☐ **B**　creatine phosphokinase
    ☐ **C**　creatinine
    ☐ **D**　daptomycin concentrations
    ☐ **E**　sodium

23 Mrs F is being managed for heart failure and her oedema has gotten worse, but her electrolyte levels are in range. The medical team decide to increase the furosemide dose from 40 mg once a day to 40 mg twice a day. Mrs F says that she will take her first dose in the morning as usual, but is not sure when to take the second dose.
What should you advise?

    ☐ **A**　At bedtime
    ☐ **B**　At lunchtime
    ☐ **C**　The prescription is incorrect and needs to go back to the prescriber
    ☐ **D**　With her evening meal
    ☐ **E**　With her morning dose

24 Mr A is a patient on your ward. Recently he has developed an acute exacerbation of gout. The medical team think that it may have been precipitated by one of his medicines.

Which one of his regular medicines do you think could have precipitated the gout?

- □ A   allopurinol
- □ B   atenolol
- □ C   bendroflumethiazide
- □ D   clopidogrel
- □ E   enalapril

25 You are on a post-take ward round with the medical team who are discussing Mr G, who currently takes *Priadel*® (lithium carbonate) 400 mg daily and zopiclone 7.5 mg at night when required. The medical team request lithium levels to confirm their diagnosis of suspected lithium toxicity.
Which of the following is NOT a sign/symptom of lithium toxicity?

- □ A   blurred vision
- □ B   convulsions
- □ C   depression
- □ D   lack of coordination
- □ E   muscle weakness

26 Mr T comes to see you at your anticoagulant clinic. You check the patient's INR and discover that it is 3.4. You read the patient's recent notes and find out that it is caused by a drug that has been recently started.
Which of the following drugs could cause an increase in the patient's INR?

- □ A   amiodarone
- □ B   carbamazepine
- □ C   phenobarbital
- □ D   rifampicin
- □ E   St John's wort

27 Mr L comes to your pharmacy complaining of a cold sore. After questioning him, you decide to sell him some aciclovir topical cream. How often should he apply the cream?

- □ A   once a day
- □ B   twice a day
- □ C   three times a day
- □ D   four times a day
- □ E   five times a day

28 Mrs U comes to your pharmacy with a prescription for acetylcysteine
5% eye drops, 1 drop into both eyes QDS; hypromellose 0.3% eye
drops, 1 drop into both eyes PRN; and levofloxacin 5 mg/mL eye
drops, 1 drop into the left eye every 4 hours for 7 days. When advising
Mrs U on how to use her eye drops, you advise her to leave a time gap
between applying each eye drop.
Which of the following is the most appropriate time interval between
eye drop applications?

    □ A   1 minute
    □ B   2 minutes
    □ C   5 minutes
    □ D   10 minutes
    □ E   No time interval is required

29 Mr Z is a 91-year-old man who has been admitted to your high
dependency unit with sepsis of unknown origin. He is confused and not
taking tablets, so he is currently receiving medicines intravenously. His
temperature is currently 38.6°C and the medical team want to prescribe
IV paracetamol to bring his temperature down. You note that Mr Z
was found to weigh 42 kg on admission.
What is the maximum dose of paracetamol that should be prescribed
for Mr Z?
You may use the paracetamol monograph in the BNF to help you
answer this question.

    □ A   420 mg
    □ B   500 mg
    □ C   630 mg
    □ D   750 mg
    □ E   1000 mg

30 Mrs E is a 36-year-old woman who is otherwise well and not taking
any other medicines. She has just been diagnosed with pneumonia and
is prescribed levofloxacin 500 mg OD and prednisolone 30 mg OD for
7 days.
Which of the following adverse reactions should Mrs E be informed of
and advised on how to identify?

    □ A   aortic aneurysm
    □ B   *Clostridium difficile* infection
    □ C   QT prolongation
    □ D   seizures
    □ E   tendon damage

31 Mrs J is a 64-year-old woman who presented to her GP complaining of dysuria, increased frequency of urination and was found to have loin tenderness. The GP diagnosed her with a lower urinary tract infection and prescribed her trimethoprim tablets 200 mg BD for 7 days. When checking her PMR you notice she had a course of trimethoprim a month ago.

Which of the following is the most appropriate course of action?

☐ A Contact the GP and advise a treatment duration of 3 days for the trimethoprim

☐ B Contact the GP and advise him/her to prescribe co-amoxiclav 500/125 mg TDS for 3 days

☐ C Contact the GP and advise him/her to prescribe fosfomycin 3 g STAT

☐ D Contact the GP and advise him/her to prescribe nitrofurantoin M/R 100 mg BD for 3 days

☐ E Dispense the prescription that has been provided

32 You are updating your local guidelines on the management of COPD and are reviewing a new clinical trial looking at exacerbation rates between patients who are prescribed fluticasone or beclometasone. Which of the following p values would indicate a statistically significant difference between these two treatments?

☐ A $p = 0.01$
☐ B $p = 0.1$
☐ C $p = 1.0$
☐ D $p = 10.0$
☐ E p values are not useful for determining differences between treatment groups

33 Miss Y has been admitted to your high dependency unit suffering from diabetic ketoacidosis, for which she is currently being given intravenous fluids and soluble insulin infused at a fix rate. When undertaking her drug history, you find Miss Y was usually taking 15 units of insulin glargine at night and variable units of insulin aspart with meals.

Which of the following is the most appropriate to do initially?

☐ A Continue with the current fluids and soluble insulin infusion regimen

☐ B Prescribe insulin glargine 13 units at night alongside the current fluids and soluble insulin infusion

☐ C Prescribe insulin glargine 15 units at night alongside the current fluids and soluble insulin infusion

> □ D   Prescribe insulin glargine 15 units at night and variable units of insulin aspart alongside the current fluids. Stop the soluble insulin infusion
> □ E   Prescribe insulin glargine 17 units at night alongside the current fluids and soluble insulin infusion

34 Mr D has been admitted to your ward after being diagnosed with severe sepsis secondary to pneumonia, for which he is being treated with co-amoxiclav and clarithromycin. Before admission, Mr D was taking methotrexate 20 mg once weekly for psoriasis.

Which of the following is the most appropriate to advise the medical team?

You may use the SPC for methotrexate tablets to help you: https://www.medicines.org.uk/emc/product/1377/smpc

> □ A   Prescribe methotrexate 10 mg once weekly whilst receiving co-amoxiclav concomitantly
> □ B   Prescribe methotrexate 20 mg once weekly, as per drug history, to prevent relapse of psoriasis
> □ C   Prescribe methotrexate 5 mg once weekly whist receiving co-amoxiclav and clarithromycin concomitantly
> □ D   Withhold methotrexate and continue current management
> □ E   Withhold methotrexate and prescribe hydrocortisone to prevent flares of psoriasis

35 Mrs W presents to your pharmacy with a prescription for 50:50 ointment to be used as a bath additive for emollient purposes.

Which of the following counselling points is the LEAST appropriate to give this patient?

> □ A   Add 50:50 ointment to bath water and use as a soak
> □ B   Apply 50:50 ointment directly to dry skin then rinse off with water
> □ C   Avoid exposure of clothing and any dressings to naked flames or cigarettes
> □ D   Can make bath and shower surfaces more slippery than normal
> □ E   Wash hands before and after using 50:50 ointment

SECTION C

Sonia Kauser

1   Mrs GS, an 82-year-old woman has been admitted onto an acute elderly medical ward in hospital due to a fall and long lie. You are the clinical pharmacist on site and have been asked to review her medication on admission. Mrs GS has informed you she has recently been initiated on a tablet but is unsure of the name or dose.
    Which of her following medication would be the most likely drug to have caused the fall?

    ☐ A   aspirin 75 mg PO OD
    ☐ B   atorvastatin 40 mg PO ON
    ☐ C   bisoprolol 2.5 mg PO OD
    ☐ D   clopidogrel 75 mg PO OD
    ☐ E   ramipril 10 mg PO OD

2   Mr GT, a 56-year-old man, attends your anticoagulation clinic for a routine warfarin appointment. He is currently being treated for stroke prevention in atrial fibrillation with a target therapeutic INR 2–3. His reading today is 3.2. He reports no side effects or bleeding and his usual dose is 5 mg daily.
    What is the most appropriate advice to this patient?

    ☐ A   Omit warfarin and recommend oral phytomenadione at 1 mg stat dose then recheck INR
    ☐ B   Omit warfarin for 1 day then return to maintenance dose of 5 mg daily and recheck INR within 7 days
    ☐ C   Omit warfarin for 3 days then return to maintenance dose of 5 mg daily and recheck INR within 7 days
    ☐ D   Reduce green vegetable intake as this will reduce INR and continue at 5 mg daily
    ☐ E   Refer to A&E as INR out of range

3   Miss KL, a 38-year-old female with known bipolar affective disorder presents to the hospital medical admissions ward with query lithium toxicity.
    Which of the following drugs from her current medication list is most likely to be the causative agent?

    ☐ A   amiodarone 200 mg PO OD
    ☐ B   bendroflumethiazide 5 mg PO OD

    ☐ C   naproxen 500 mg PO BD
    ☐ D   paracetamol 1 g PO QDS
    ☐ E   sodium valproate 200 mg PO BD

4   You are a prescribing pharmacist working within a local GP surgery. You are required to undertake a medication review for Mrs SN, a 54-year-old woman. You note that one of her medications can prolong the QT interval. Which of the following drugs do you decide to review?

    ☐ A   bendroflumethiazide 2.5 mg PO OM
    ☐ B   citalopram 30 mg PO OD
    ☐ C   levothyroxine 25 mcg PO OD
    ☐ D   mirtazapine 45 mg PO ON
    ☐ E   naproxen 250 mg PO BD

5   Mr BH, a 67-year-old man has been admitted into hospital due to AKI. Which of the following medication is the likely causative agent?

    ☐ A   bendroflumethiazide 5 mg OD
    ☐ B   furosemide 40 mg OD
    ☐ C   ramipril 5 mg OD
    ☐ D   rivaroxaban 20 mg OD
    ☐ E   simvastatin 40 mg ON

6   Which of the following medication should be prescribed by brand due to differences in bioavailability between various formulations?

    ☐ A   apixaban
    ☐ B   digoxin
    ☐ C   diltiazem S/R
    ☐ D   metformin M/R
    ☐ E   venlafaxine M/R

7   You are a prescribing pharmacist managing a type 2 diabetes clinic. Mrs KS, a 47-year-old female, presents to your clinic with sweating, headache and nausea. You are able to check her blood glucose and it is currently 2.9 mmol/L.
What may have caused these symptoms and the reading to arise?

    ☐ A   alogliptin 25 mg OD
    ☐ B   bisoprolol 10 mg OD
    ☐ C   clopidogrel 75 mg OD
    ☐ D   metformin M/R 1 g TDS
    ☐ E   recent weight gain

8   Mr DT, a 52-year-old man presents to the community pharmacy with persistent and severe abdominal pain which has recently started. You access his PMR and note he is prescribed the following medication:

- alogliptin 25 mg OD (started 1 month ago)
- metformin 500 mg BD (started 2 months ago)
- aspirin 75 mg OD (started 8 years ago)
- ranitidine 150 mg BD (started 3 years ago)
- ramipril 5 mg OD (started 8 years ago)

- citalopram 20 mg OD (started 1 year ago)
- codeine 30 mg up to QDS PRN
- atorvastatin 40 mg ON (started 8 years ago)
- bisoprolol 5 mg OD (started 8 years ago)

Which of the following is the most appropriate advice to give to Mr DT?

- ☐ **A**   Stop alogliptin and urgent referral to GP
- ☐ **B**   Stop aspirin and urgent referral to GP
- ☐ **C**   Stop citalopram and urgent referral to GP
- ☐ **D**   Stop codeine and urgent referral to GP
- ☐ **E**   Stop metformin and urgent referral to GP

9   Mr GS, aged 62, visits your community pharmacy and is requesting treatment for oral thrush. He recalls "using some sort of topical preparation" in the past but is unsure what was issued. He has no known allergies and his PMR shows he is prescribed the following medication: amlodipine 5 mg OD, levothyroxine 125 mg OD, atorvastatin 20 mg OD, warfarin 3 mg OD, lansoprazole 15 mg OD.
How do you manage this patient?

- ☐ **A**   Refer to GP
- ☐ **B**   Supply OTC anbesol liquid gel
- ☐ **C**   Supply OTC benzydamine 15% spray
- ☐ **D**   Supply OTC miconazole gel
- ☐ **E**   Supply OTC *Orajel*®

10 Mr IK, aged 55, has recently been diagnosed with an acute ischaemic stroke following discharge from hospital.
What is the likely combination that he will be prescribed with?

- ☐ **A**   Aspirin PO 150 mg daily for 2 weeks then long term antiplatelet therapy

☐ B   Aspirin PO 150 mg daily for 3 weeks then long term antiplatelet therapy

☐ C   Aspirin PO 150 mg daily for 4 weeks then long term antiplatelet therapy

☐ D   Aspirin PO 300 mg daily for 2 weeks then long term antiplatelet therapy

☐ E   Aspirin PO 300 mg daily for 3 weeks then long term antiplatelet therapy

11 Mrs GS has been diagnosed with non-valvular atrial fibrillation and has been initiated on apixaban 2.5 mg PO BD to prevent stroke or systemic embolic events.

What one of the following is a correct statement regarding baseline monitoring requirements?

☐ A   Blood pressure, full blood count, liver function tests, urea and electrolytes

☐ B   Blood pressure, full blood count, urea and electrolytes

☐ C   Blood pressure, QRISK score, serum creatinine, urea and electrolytes

☐ D   Body weight, serum creatinine, urea and electrolytes

☐ E   Body weight, serum creatinine, urea and electrolytes, liver function tests, full blood count

12 Mr FN, aged 82, has been admitted into hospital due to drowsiness and confusion. The reading from his bloods are as follows:

- K = 4.2
- Na = 120
- eGFR = 70 mL/min

Which of his regular medication is the most likely agent to have contributed to his symptoms and the recent results?

☐ A   codeine 15 mg up to PO QDS PRN
☐ B   ramipril 5 mg PO OD
☐ C   ranitidine 300 mg PO OD
☐ D   rivaroxaban 15 mg PO OD
☐ E   sertraline 100 mg PO OD

13 Miss SR, a 28-year-old female presents to the pharmacy with a prescription for isotretinoin. She is currently under the Pregnancy Prevention Programme (PPP) and has previously tolerated this medication. Under the PPP, how long is this prescription valid for?

☐ A   7 days
☐ B   14 days

    ☐ C   21 days
    ☐ D   28 days
    ☐ E   6 months

14 Mrs AB, aged 42, has been initiated on amiodarone for the treatment of arrhythmias.
Which of the following statements is correct regarding the baseline monitoring that is required?

    ☐ A   Chest X-ray, blood pressure, weight, full blood count
    ☐ B   Chest X-ray, thyroid function tests, liver function tests, serum potassium
    ☐ C   ECG, chest X-ray, blood pressure, urea and electrolytes
    ☐ D   ECG, full blood count, thyroid function tests
    ☐ E   ECG, liver function tests, blood pressure

15 Mrs GT, aged 59, visits your community pharmacy and complains of muscular aches and pains in both legs.
Which medication is associated with potentially serious side effects?

    ☐ A   amitriptyline 50 mg ON
    ☐ B   naproxen 500 mg BD
    ☐ C   quetiapine 400 mg M/R ON
    ☐ D   quinine 200 mg ON
    ☐ E   simvastatin 40 mg ON

16 Mr FN, aged 73, has a QRISK score of 15%. His current medication are as follows: amlodipine 5 mg, fluoxetine 20 mg OD, *Gaviscon Advance®* 5–10 mLs PRN, naproxen 250 mg BD PRN, lansoprazole 15 mg OD.
What do you recommend as an appropriate course of action?

    ☐ A   Recheck QRISK in 12 months as score is <20% therefore no further action required
    ☐ B   Recommend atorvastatin 10 mg OD due to interaction with amlodipine
    ☐ C   Recommend atorvastatin 20 mg ON
    ☐ D   Recommend simvastatin 20 mg ON due to interaction with amlodipine
    ☐ E   Recommend simvastatin 40 mg ON

17 A GP contacts you regarding appropriate antibiotic treatment for an 11-year-old with a respiratory infection. You note from the records you have access to that the patient is allergic to penicillin.

What is the appropriate treatment recommendation?

    □ A   amoxicillin 250 mg TDS for 7 days
    □ B   ciprofloxacin 250 mg BD for 7 days
    □ C   co-amoxiclav 250/125 mg TDS for 7 days
    □ D   doxycycline 100 mg OD for 7 days
    □ E   erythromycin 250 mg QDS for 7 days

18 Mrs SR, aged 78, has been diagnosed with an uncomplicated lower urinary tract infection. Her eGFR is 45 mL/min. She has no known drug allergies.
Her current medication is as follows: paracetamol 1g PO QDS, Calceos® 1 BD, methotrexate 7.5 mg once weekly, folic acid 5 mg every day (except for the day of methotrexate), pantoprazole 20 mg OD, piroxicam gel 0.5% topical TDS, amlodipine 5 mg daily.
What antibiotic treatment do you recommend?

    □ A   nitrofurantoin 50 mg QDS for 3 days
    □ B   pivmecillinam initially 400 mg for 1 dose then 200 mg TDS for 3 days
    □ C   pivmecillinam initially 400 mg for 1 dose then 200 mg TDS for 7 days
    □ D   trimethoprim 200 mg BD for 3 days
    □ E   trimethoprim 200 mg BD for 7 days

19 Which of the following antidepressant medications is associated with the most withdrawal side effects if stopped abruptly?

    □ A   citalopram 20 mg OD
    □ B   escitalopram 20 mg OD
    □ C   fluoxetine 20 mg OD
    □ D   fluoxetine 60 mg OD
    □ E   paroxetine 40 mg OD

20 Mrs SB, aged 32, has recently been diagnosed with mild depression. She has no other co-morbidities but in the past has attempted suicide. Which of the following antidepressant medications should be AVOIDED due to the increased risk of fatality in overdose?

    □ A   amitriptyline 200 mg ON
    □ B   lofepramine 140 mg ON
    □ C   mirtazapine 45 mg ON
    □ D   paroxetine 20 mg OD
    □ E   trazodone 300 mg ON

21 Miss SM, a 23-year-old female visits your pharmacy as she is requesting the emergency contraceptive pill. You decide to undertake a consultation (within a private area) and note that the unprotected sexual intercourse took place 74 hours ago. She takes no other prescribed medication and has no other medical conditions.

What do you recommend?

☐ A levonorgestrel 1.5 mg PO Stat
☐ B levonorgestrel 3 mg PO Stat
☐ C refer to GP
☐ D ulipristal acetate 30 mg PO Stat
☐ E ulipristal acetate 60 mg PO Stat

22 Miss SK, a 58-year-old woman visits your community pharmacy for a routine blood pressure check. Her comorbidities include hypertension and diabetes.

What is her target blood pressure that you will be assessing?

☐ A 120/80
☐ B 130/80
☐ C 140/80
☐ D 140/90
☐ E 150/90

23 Miss HA, aged 32, has been initiated on an acute course of steroid for an exacerbation of asthma (prednisolone 40 mg PO OD for 5 days). Which of the following is a side effect associated with steroids?

☐ A hyperglycaemia
☐ B hypernatraemia
☐ C hyponatraemia
☐ D hypotension
☐ E weight loss

24 Miss RK, aged 42, has been initiated on methotrexate PO 10 mg weekly for rheumatoid arthritis. Which of the following are essential monitoring parameters (baseline and routine)?

☐ A BP, liver function tests, ECG
☐ B ECG, urea and electrolytes, full blood count
☐ C Liver function tests, creatinine, full blood count
☐ D No routine monitoring needed
☐ E Serum drug levels, full blood count, BP

25 Miss FT, aged 57, is currently being managed for her type 2 diabetes. Her current medication is metformin 1 g BD, gliclazide 80 mg BD, furosemide 20 mg OD, ramipril 2.5 mg OD. Her diabetes nurse has decided not to initiate her on pioglitazone due to risks associated. Which of the following statements is correct with regards to pioglitazone?

  □ A   Avoid prescribing alongside metformin
  □ B   Dose of concomitant sulfonylurea may need to be increased
  □ C   Pioglitazone should not be used in patients with heart failure or a past medical history of heart failure
  □ D   Review treatment after 12 months of initiation
  □ E   There is a high risk of bladder cancer and should be avoided even in those who respond adequately to treatment

26 Which of the following medication requires female patients of child-bearing potential to agree NOT to fall pregnant (as per the Pregnancy Prevention Programme) whilst taking this medication due to risk of birth defects?

  □ A   dalteparin
  □ B   diclofenac
  □ C   glibenclamide
  □ D   levothyroxine
  □ E   sodium valproate

27 Which of the following is a common side effect associated with amlodipine?

  □ A   gastro-intestinal disturbances
  □ B   hypotension
  □ C   muscle cramps
  □ D   oedema
  □ E   paraesthesia

28 Miss KL, aged 22, presents to your pharmacy with a headache due to stress related to her exam revision. The headache has the following characteristics: pulsating in character, unilateral pain, feeling nauseaous. This headache started 6 hours ago and she notices that there has been a trend for these headaches (they occur if she misses a meal, has a high caffeine intake or is feeling stressed). She has no allergies, is taking no medication and has no other medical conditions.
What is the appropriate way to manage this patient?

  □ A   Advise no analgesia or medication needed currently
  □ B   Migraine diagnosis – offer sumatriptan OTC as pharmacist can also diagnose

☐ C   Migraine diagnosis – refer to GP for sumatriptan as a GP can only diagnose this

☐ D   Tension type headache – offer OTC analgesia such as paracetamol or ibuprofen

☐ E   Tension type headache – refer to GP for further management

29   Mrs AB, a 56-year-old woman has been prescribed HRT therapy – *Elleste duet*® 1 mg daily. She visits your pharmacy and informs you she is worried about the side effects.

Which of the following statements is INCORRECT with regards to her HRT therapy?

☐ A   The medication will be taken in cyclical form, Mrs AB will take for 21 days and have a 7 day break

☐ B   There is an increased breast cancer risk with this therapy

☐ C   There is an increased endometrial cancer risk

☐ D   There is an increased ovarian cancer risk

☐ E   Women who are already prescribed anticoagulation therapy need careful consideration of the benefits versus risks of HRT use due to VTE risk

30   You are a community pharmacist working in a health centre. The pharmacy is based next door to a medical practice. You are contacted by a relevant prescriber (doctor) who is requesting an emergency supply of tramadol 100 mg M/R capsules for a patient who has osteoarthritis and is requiring urgent pain relief.

Which of the following is a correct statement regarding this request?

☐ A   Can be supplied provided the doctor provides an indication to the nature of the emergency and the prescription is received within 48 hours

☐ B   Can be supplied provided the written prescription is received within 72 hours

☐ C   Can be supplied provided the written prescription is received within 48 hours

☐ D   Cannot be supplied as tramadol is not permitted for emergency supplies

☐ E   Cannot be supplied as you are based in a health centre and there is access to a surgery

31   Mr DT, a 52-year-old man is prescribed sildenafil at a dose of 50 mg prior to sexual intercourse (indication – erectile dysfunction). He presents to your pharmacy with his prescription. This is the first

time he is taking this medication and after reviewing his PMR you decide to consult with him (GTN spray prescribed for stable angina). Which of the following is the most appropriate counselling?

- ☐ **A** No counselling required
- ☐ **B** Sildenafil is contraindicated in stable angina, refer to GP
- ☐ **C** Take once a day approximately 2 hours before sexual activity
- ☐ **D** This combination should be avoided with a GTN spray. Do not use at the same time as a GTN spray due to increased risk of hypotension
- ☐ **E** This dose can be taken more than once per day

32 A palliative care nurse requests your advice regarding a patient who is end of life. The plan is to amend the current PO medication to SC administration. The patient is currently prescribed 60 mg M/R BD and takes 2.5 mLs of breakthrough pain relief (*Oramorph*® 10 mg/5 mL) four times a day.
What will you recommend as the S/C dose over 24 hours?

- ☐ **A** 65 mg S/C over 24 hours
- ☐ **B** 70 mg S/C over 24 hours
- ☐ **C** 120 mg S/C over 24 hours
- ☐ **D** 130 mg S/C over 24 hours
- ☐ **E** 140 mg S/C over 24 hours

33 Mrs KC presents to the community pharmacy with her son, who is 2-years-old, requesting treatment for his eye. You consult with this patient and Mrs KC and note the following symptoms: one eye affected, no pain, excessive discharge in the morning, vision unaffected.
How do you manage this patient?

- ☐ **A** Offer chloramphenicol 0.5% eye drops
- ☐ **B** Offer sodium chloride ophthalmic eye drops to rinse the eye
- ☐ **C** Offer sodium cromoglycate 2% eye drops
- ☐ **D** Recommend lid hygiene
- ☐ **E** Refer to GP as no product available for this age

34 Mrs GK, a 52-year-old female of Afro-Caribbean descent, has been diagnosed with hypertension due to recent elevated blood pressure readings (most recent reading is 155/92). You have been asked by the multidisciplinary team to recommend an appropriate antihypertensive. What do you recommend?

- ☐ **A** amlodipine 5 mg OD
- ☐ **B** candesartan 8 mg OD

☐ C   enalapril 5 mg OD
☐ D   ramipril 1.25 mg OD
☐ E   ramipril 10 mg OD

35 Mrs TB, aged 62, visits your pharmacy to collect her medication. She has recently been prescribed doxycycline capsules 100 mg OD for 7 days and this is the first time she will be taking her medication. Which of the following is the INCORRECT advice for this patient?

☐ A   Do not take indigestion remedies, or medicines containing iron or zinc, 2 hours before or after you take this medicine
☐ B   Protect your skin from sunlight – even on a bright but cloudy day. Do not use sunbeds
☐ C   Space the doses evenly throughout the day. Keep taking this medicine until the course is finished, unless you are told to stop
☐ D   Take with a full glass of water
☐ E   This medicine may colour your urine – this is harmless

36 Which of the following statements is INCORRECT with regards to the New Medicines Service (NMS)?

☐ A   The medicines list for NMS condition therapy areas includes antiplatelet/anticoagulant therapy
☐ B   The medicines list for NMS condition therapy areas includes asthma and COPD
☐ C   The medicines list for NMS condition therapy areas includes hypertension
☐ D   The medicines list for NMS condition therapy areas includes patients taking high risk medication
☐ E   The medicines list for NMS condition therapy areas includes type 2 diabetes

37 Mr ZB, aged 33, attends the community pharmacy and requests *Gaviscon*® liquid for relief of his heart burn. Upon questioning you note he is currently taking the following medication: paracetamol 500 mg QDS PRN, ferrous sulphate 200 mg TDS and citalopram 10 mg daily. What is the most appropriate advice to give to this patient with regards to his request for antacid medication?

☐ A   Antacids decrease the absorption of iron therefore iron should be taken 1 hour before the antacid or 2 hours after the antacid
☐ B   Antacids decrease the absorption of iron therefore iron should be taken on an empty stomach to promote absorption

☐ C   Iron decreases the absorption of antacids therefore iron should be taken 1 hour before the antacid or 2 hours after the antacid

☐ D   Iron decreases the absorption of antacids therefore iron should be taken on an empty stomach to promote absorption

☐ E   There is no interaction between antacids and iron medication therefore both can be taken at the same time

38 Mrs SM, aged 62, attends the community pharmacy and informs you she has recently developed "a tingling sensation" in her hands and feet and on certain occasions notices cold extremities in her hands. She reports no other symptoms and has no pain. You check her medication record and are able to note that one of her tablets may be the cause of this symptom.

Which of the following medication is the most likely to be the cause?

☐ A   aspirin
☐ B   bisoprolol
☐ C   empagliflozin
☐ D   ramipril
☐ E   spironolactone

39 Mrs FR, aged 54, attends your pharmacy and is supplied with an acute supply of prednisolone tablets (short 2-week course) as directed by her respiratory specialist. You check her past medical record and are able to note she has the following conditions: diabetes mellitus, COPD, atrial fibrillation.

What would be the most appropriate advice to give to this patient?

☐ A   Measure blood pressure (BP) and pulse due to possibilities of increased pulse rate

☐ B   Measure blood pressure (BP) and pulse due to possibilities of reduced pulse rate

☐ C   Monitor forced vital capacity (FVC) until course complete

☐ D   Undertake blood glucose monitoring due to risk of hyperglycaemia

☐ E   Undertake blood glucose monitoring due to risk of hypoglycaemia

40 Mrs JK, a 68-year-old woman has been initiated on alendronic acid 70 mg once weekly therapy for the primary prevention of osteoporotic fractures (she has confirmed osteoporosis). She presents her prescription to the pharmacy and is querying the treatment duration of her medication.

Which of the following statements is correct?

- [ ] **A** The need to continue treatment after re-evaluation based on assessment of risks versus benefits, tends to be long term
- [ ] **B** The need to continue treatment should be re-evaluated periodically based on assessment of risks versus benefits
- [ ] **C** The need to continue treatment should be re-evaluated periodically based on assessment of risks versus benefits, particularly after 5 years or more
- [ ] **D** The need to continue treatment should be re-evaluated periodically based on assessment of risks versus benefits, particularly after 2 years or more
- [ ] **E** The need to continue treatment should be re-evaluated periodically based on assessment of risks versus benefits, particularly after 4 years or more

41 Miss AK, aged 23, visits your pharmacy with a prescription for desogestrel 75 mcg once daily. This is the first time she is administering an oral contraceptive pill. You decide to counsel her on her new medication. Which of the following statements is true with regards to progesterone only contraceptives?

- [ ] **A** Clinical trials have demonstrated progesterone only contraceptive is more effective than combined hormonal contraceptives.
- [ ] **B** It is a suitable alternative where oestrogens are contraindicated (such as history of migraine with aura)
- [ ] **C** It is not a suitable alternative to combined hormonal contraceptives where oestrogens are contraindicated
- [ ] **D** Take one daily for 21 days then stop taking for 7 days (pill-free break)
- [ ] **E** Vomiting and persistent diarrhoea does not affect the absorption of the progesterone only contraceptive

42 Mr AK, aged 56, presents to your pharmacy with a new prescription – finasteride 5 mg tablets once daily – for benign prostatic hyperplasia. What appropriate counselling should be given to this patient according to MHRA/CDM advice?

- [ ] **A** Breast enlargement can occur, stop taking the finasteride if this occurs
- [ ] **B** Depression can occur; stop taking finasteride if this occurs and seek advice from a healthcare professional

    ☐ C   Review treatment at 12 months before considering long-term use

    ☐ D   This medication can cause male pattern hair loss, stop taking this medication if this occurs

    ☐ E   This medication can cause testicular cancer

43 Mrs TB presents with a veterinary prescription to your pharmacy at the request for medication to be supplied under the cascade system. This request is for Tom, the dog.

    Which of the following is NOT a legal requirement on the prescription?

    ☐ A   Address of prescriber
    ☐ B   Date of birth of animal
    ☐ C   Dose of medication
    ☐ D   Identity and species of animal
    ☐ E   Telephone number of prescriber

44 Mrs SA, aged 54, is prescribed clozapine for the management of schizophrenia.

    Which of the following is NOT part of the long term monitoring requirements?

    ☐ A   blood counts including leucocytes
    ☐ B   blood glucose levels
    ☐ C   blood pressure
    ☐ D   lipids
    ☐ E   weight

45 Mrs DT, aged 56, has been initiated on warfarin therapy due to a recent onset of atrial fibrillation.

    Which of the following is an appropriate tool used to assess which patients should be initiated on this therapy?

    ☐ A CHA_2DS_2VASC Score
    ☐ B   Glasgow-Blatchford bleeding score
    ☐ C   HAS-BLED Score
    ☐ D   NYHA classification
    ☐ E   QRISK Score

SECTION D

Oksana Pyzik

1   Ms UX, a 60-year-old female with Parkinson's disease is admitted to hospital and presents with severe nausea. The prescriber orders a blood test which shows low levels of potassium at 2.2 mmol/L and normal levels of creatinine, urea and sodium.
Which of the following medicines on Ms UX's drug chart would you recommend to the prescriber to STOP immediately?

   ☐ A   bendroflumethiazide
   ☐ B   bisoprolol
   ☐ C   cyclizine
   ☐ D   domperidone
   ☐ E   lisinopril

2   A 40-year-old woman asks to speak to the pharmacist about her family history of breast cancer.
Which one of the following statements is INCORRECT around genetic predisposition of breast cancer?

   ☐ A   Refer directly to a specialist genetics service if a high-risk predisposing gene mutation has been identified
   ☐ B   The majority of increase in risk of breast cancer is due to the presence of gene mutations such as BRCA1, BRCA2 or TP53
   ☐ C   The risk of breast cancer in women with an affected first-degree relative is approximately twice the risk in other women
   ☐ D   The risk of breast cancer increases as the age of affected relatives decreases
   ☐ E   The risk of breast cancer increases with the number of affected relatives

3   A 46-year-old male with a history of ulcerative colitis presents at the hospital complaining of severe indigestion pain for the past 4 weeks. Upon further physical examination the pain was identified in the region of the central abdomen lying below the sternum and above the umbilicus.
Which one of the following medicines is most likely to be linked to the epigastric pain?

   ☐ A   atenolol
   ☐ B   baclofen

☐ C   mesalazine
☐ D   olanzapine
☐ E   prednisolone

4   A 76-year-old women with a history of hypertension and osteoarthritis is hospitalised due to shortness of breath, severe oedema and decreased urine output. Her blood test results are as follows:

	Value	Normal range
Na (mmol/L)	137	135–145
K (mmol/L)	5.2	3.5–5.0
Ur (mmol/L)	14	3–7
Cr (µmol/L)	243	60–125

The prescriber believes the symptoms may be linked to her medicines. Which one of the following medicines would you recommend to the prescriber to STOP immediately?

☐ A   alendronic acid 70 mg once weekly
☐ B   calcium carbonate (1500 mg) and vitamin D_3 (400 I.U.) OD
☐ C   paracetamol 500 mg QDS
☐ D   prednisolone 30 mg OD
☐ E   ramipril 5 mg OD

5   A 45-year-old male is diagnosed with androgenic alopecia.
Which of the following medicines is the most appropriate for this patient?

☐ A   dutasteride 500 mcg tablets
☐ B   finasteride 1 mg tablets
☐ C   minoxidil 5 mg tablets
☐ D   tadalafil 20 mg tablets
☐ E   tamsulosin 400 mcg tablets

6   A 25-year-old woman who suffers from epilepsy is trying to get pregnant.
What dose of folic acid should she be prescribed?

☐ A   5 mg
☐ B   20 mg
☐ C   40 mg
☐ D   400 mcg
☐ E   1000 mcg

7 A 67-year-old male with a history of myocardial infarction and atrial fibrillation, is currently taking 3 mg of warfarin and 5 mg of ramipril daily. He presents at the anticoagulant clinic to monitor his INR. He appears well with no signs of bleeding and the tests reveal an INR of 6.2 (target 2–3). He was treated for a respiratory infection seven days ago with a course of clarithromycin.

Which one of the following actions is most appropriate for the prescriber to take?

□ A   Administer 5 mg vitamin K IV
□ B   Increase next dose of warfarin
□ C   Omit warfarin and recheck INR
□ D   Reduce next dose of warfarin
□ E   Stop ramipril 5 mg

8 Which one of the following statements with regards to withdrawing anti-epileptic therapy is correct?

□ A   The decision to withdraw should be taken primarily by the specialist
□ B   The patient must be seizure-free for at least 5 years
□ C   Withdraw antiepileptic drugs gradually over a period of 4–6 weeks
□ D   Withdraw benzodiazepines over a period of 2–3 months
□ E   Withdraw one drug at a time if on multiple regime

9 A 50-year-old male presents with hypo-pigmented macules and patches on his left arm and upper back which are slightly pink in colour and covered in a fine powdery scale. Upon further questioning you discover that the patches are not painful and have not spread further.

Which one of the following is the most likely diagnosis for this patient?

□ A   eczema
□ B   pityriasis versicolor
□ C   psoriasis
□ D   rosacea
□ E   vitiligo

10 A 34-year-old male is started on citalopram for depression alongside cognitive behavioural therapy. He is due for a check-up in two weeks' time with the GP. Which one of the following is the most appropriate to monitor for this patient?

□ A   Assess for efficacy
□ B   Assess for signs of suicidal ideation

    ☐ C   Blood Pressure
    ☐ D   Echocardiogram
    ☐ E   Full blood count

11 A 32-year-old female suffers from migraines and is prescribed pro-
    pranolol for prophylaxis. However, she is uncomfortable taking pro-
    pranolol daily and would like to avoid taking any medicines at all if
    possible. She asks the pharmacist about the side effects of propranolol
    to help inform her decision.
    Which one of the following is a common side effect of propanolol?

    ☐ A   anhidrosis
    ☐ B   anxiety
    ☐ C   fatigue
    ☐ D   syncopye
    ☐ E   tachycardia

12 An 85-year-old male frequently calls the pharmacy to verify his daily
    dose of simvastatin. He is taking 13 different medications and does not
    have a carer. He calls again today to ask the same question.
    Which one of the following actions would you take as the pharmacist?

    ☐ A   Answer his question and call the GP to suggest switching to
          another statin
    ☐ B   Answer his question and suggest that the patient make a
          note of the answer
    ☐ C   Answer his question and suggest that the pharmacy create a
          blister pack for the patient to keep track
    ☐ D   Call the GP and suggest that the patient be transferred into
          a nursing home
    ☐ E   Suggest that the labels are printed with a larger font

13 A 73-year-old female inpatient in hospital is diagnosed with a severe
    urinary tract infection. Her baseline creatinine levels upon admission
    were recorded at 93 μmol/L and by day 4 rose to 193 μmol/L. The
    patient has had plenty of fluids and has no previous history of renal
    impairment. She is taking ramipril alongside the medicines listed below.
    Which one of the following medicines is most likely to have caused a
    decline in renal function for this patient?

    ☐ A   amlodipine
    ☐ B   codeine phosphate
    ☐ C   diclofenac
    ☐ D   nitrofurantoin
    ☐ E   selegline

14 A 65-year-old female has been admitted to hospital for knee surgery. She has a history of rheumatoid arthritis and is taking methotrexate. Upon admission she also develops a urinary tract infection and is treated with antibiotics. A blood test reveals that her neutrophil count is declining.
Which one of the following medicines is most likely to have caused the neutropenia?

    □ A   aspirin
    □ B   bendroflumethiazide
    □ C   gabapentin
    □ D   prednisolone
    □ E   trimethoprim

15 A 55-year-old women with diabetes is taking insulin. She presents at the pharmacy confused and dizzy and her blood glucose reading is at 3 mmol/L.
Which one of the following is the most appropriate action to take?

    □ A   Call 999
    □ B   Give 4–5 dextrose tablets and retest blood glucose in 15 minutes
    □ C   Refer to A&E
    □ D   Retest blood glucose in one hour and report results to GP
    □ E   Suggest a carbohydrate rich meal and retest blood glucose in 1 hour

16 A 36-year-old male who is taking carbimazole for the treatment of thyrotocixosis complains of a sore throat.
Which one of the following test results would be most important in this case?

    □ A   blood cultures
    □ B   C reactive protein
    □ C   neutrophil count
    □ D   throat swab
    □ E   thyroid stimulating hormone

17 A 37-year-old female was admitted to hospital for stroke and was prescribed simvastatin 40 mg alongside other medicines for secondary prevention.
Which one of the following is the most appropriate advice to give this patient?

    □ A   Increase dose of simvastatin if muscle cramps develop
    □ B   Simvastatin is most effective in the morning

   ☐ C   Simvastatin is safe to use in active liver disease
   ☐ D   Stop treatment during pregnancy
   ☐ E   There are no dietary restrictions with statin therapy

18 A 58-year-old has been diagnosed with lung cancer and has a poor prognosis.
Which one of the following is the LEAST appropriate action to take as a pharmacist?

   ☐ A   Allow the patient to cry
   ☐ B   Answer the patient's questions about alternative therapies
   ☐ C   Calm the patient down and invite patient to discuss concerns in the consultation room
   ☐ D   Discuss the various support groups available to the patient
   ☐ E   Tell the patient that everything is going to be ok

19 A 79-year-old female weighing 78 kg has been diagnosed with hypothyroidism and is initiated on low dose levothyroxine. She has a history of type 2 diabetes and chronic stable angina and is taking metformin and GTN spray PRN.
Which one of the following is the most appropriate rationale for starting the patient on low dose thyroxine?

   ☐ A   age
   ☐ B   diabetes
   ☐ C   drug interaction
   ☐ D   gender
   ☐ E   weight

20 Which one of the following statements is LEAST aligned with principles of prescribing treatments for infectious diseases?

   ☐ A   Avoid narrow spectrum antibiotics where broad-spectrum antibiotics remain effective
   ☐ B   Avoid widespread use of topical antibiotics
   ☐ C   Consider delayed prescribing for urinary tract infections
   ☐ D   In pregnancy take specimens to inform treatment, where possible avoid tetracycline, aminoglycosides and quinolones
   ☐ E   Limit prescribing over the telephone to exceptional cases

21 A 51-year-old male has been diagnosed with Cushing's syndrome after tests revealed high levels of free cortisol in the patient's urine.
Which one of the following medicines is used as a diagnostic to assess adrenal gland function?

   ☐ A   budesonide
   ☐ B   dexamethasone

☐ C   prednisolone
☐ D   spironolactone
☐ E   triamcinolone acetonide

22 A 22-year-old male with asthma has been using a salbutamol 100 mcg inhaler (2 puffs BD) since being diagnosed with asthma 3 months ago. He complains of tremor and worsening night time cough, but reports that increased use of his inhaler has helped with reducing the frequency of coughing. You test his peak expiratory flow which has dropped by 15% since the last assessment.
Which one of the following is the most appropriate treatment option for this patient?

☐ A   Add beclometasone 200 mcg, 1 puff BD inhaled
☐ B   Add prednisolone 20 mg daily for 21 days
☐ C   Counsel on salbutamol overuse and add inhaled steroid
☐ D   Increase salbutamol inhaler to 4 puffs BD
☐ E   Stop salbutamol 100 mcg inhaler

23 A 16-month-old boy develops cold-like symptoms and a barking cough. Over a 48-hour period his symptoms worsen, with rasping noises upon inhalation and overall strenuous breathing.
Which one of the following treatment options is most appropriate in this case?

☐ A   amoxicillin
☐ B   dexamathesone
☐ C   ibuprofen
☐ D   paracetamol
☐ E   phenoxymethylpenicillin

24 A 24-year-old male was diagnosed with schizophrenia 5 years ago. He was initiated on risperidone for 2 years before switching to quetiapine 12 months ago. Recently his symptoms have worsened and the prescriber consults with you about changing his treatment to clozapine.
Which one of the following statements is most appropriate for you to discuss with the prescriber?

☐ A   Clozapine is appropriate because it has the safest side effect profile
☐ B   Clozapine is appropriate because it may help patients who fail on other antipsychotics
☐ C   Clozapine is appropriate only if given as an adjunct to quetiapine

☐ **D** Clozapine is not appropriate because it will likely produce the same effect as quietiapine

☐ **E** Clozapine is not appropriate because the risk of adverse effects is too high

25 A 55-year-old woman with breast cancer has had a total mastectomy. She has been prescribed tamoxifen 20 mg for positive oestrogen receptors on the tumour. She is currently taking warfarin, propranolol and metformin daily.

Which one of the following counselling points is the LEAST appropriate advice to give?

☐ **A** May cause hot flushes
☐ **B** Report irregular vaginal bleeding
☐ **C** Report to hospital immediately if there is any redness, pain or swelling of the leg
☐ **D** Take once weekly
☐ **E** Tamoxifen interacts with warfarin as it increases its efficacy

26 An 86-year-old man is receiving palliative care for pancreatic cancer and has been prescribed morphine sulphate 200 mg capsule BD to relieve pain. He is immobile and has had trouble eating and drinking and is slightly dehydrated.

Which one of the following medicines may predispose to faecal impaction in this patient?

☐ **A** bisacodyl
☐ **B** co-danthramer
☐ **C** ispaghula husk
☐ **D** lactulose
☐ **E** loperamide

27 A 27-year-old female is undergoing routine screening for cervical cancer and asks what are the signs and symptoms of cervical cancer.

Which one of the following symptoms is LEAST likely to be associated with cervical cancer?

☐ **A** hirsutism
☐ **B** hydronephrosis
☐ **C** irregular vaginal bleeding
☐ **D** unexplained, persistent back pain
☐ **E** unexplained, persistent pelvic pain

Questions 28 and 29 refer to Mrs NM, a 78-year-old female diagnosed with Parkinson's disease 8 years ago and is currently taking the following medicines:

- alendronic acid 70 mg once weekly
- bisprolol 2.5 mg OD
- calcium citrate 500 mg TDS
- levodopa-carbidopa CR 200/50 mg BD
- furosemide 20 mg OD
- donepezil 10 mg OD
- risperidone 0.5 mg BD
- simvastatin 40 mg ON

28 Mrs NM complains of frequent night time waking due to increased urgency to urinate.
Which one of the following medicines is most likely contributing to Mrs NM's urinary incontinence?

    ☐ A   alendronic acid
    ☐ B   donepezil
    ☐ C   furesomide
    ☐ D   levodopa-carbidopa
    ☐ E   simvastatin

29 Which one of the following medicines may further exacerbate the symptoms of Parkinson's disease?

    ☐ A   alendronic acid
    ☐ B   calcium citrate
    ☐ C   donepezil
    ☐ D   risperidone
    ☐ E   simvastatin

30 A 50-year-old male is diagnosed with congestive heart failure. He also suffers from type 2 diabetes and has mild hypertension. He suffered a mild stroke last year as a result of non-valvular atrial fibrillation.
Which one of the following anticoagulants would you prescribe for this patient?

    ☐ A   acenocoumarol
    ☐ B   apixaban
    ☐ C   aspirin
    ☐ D   phenindone
    ☐ E   warfarin

31 A 61-year-old female is diagnosed with arrhythmia and is prescribed oral amiodarone. She is started on 200 mg TDS for 1 week and reduced to 200 mg BD for a further week and then reduced again to 200 mg OD as a maintenance dose.

Which one of the following is correct with regards to this patient's treatment plan?

    □ A   A baseline chest X-ray should be conducted before starting therapy

    □ B   Administer with caution in patients with hyperkalaemia

    □ C   Liver function should be checked at baseline and repeated during therapy only if hepatotoxicity is suspected.

    □ D   May cause irreversible corneal microdeposits in the eye

    □ E   Serum creatinine should be measured before starting therapy

32 A 42-year-old female is diagnosed with thyrotoxicosis and is prescribed carbimazole as part of a 'block and replace' regimen. You counsel the patient that she should seek immediate medical attention if she develops a sore throat.

Which one of the following would be most appropriate to check first in a patient that presents with a sore throat and is taking carbimazole?

    □ A   erythrocyte sedimentation rate

    □ B   neutrophil count

    □ C   serum alanine aminotransferase

    □ D   throat swab

    □ E   thyroid function tests

33 A 43-year-old male of Caucasian descent is diagnosed with stage 1 hypertension. He weighs 108 kg and is 190 cm tall.

Which one of the following parameters should be tested before commencing treatment with ramipril?

    □ A   full blood count

    □ B   serum alanine aminotransferase

    □ C   serum creatinine

    □ D   serum glucose

    □ E   white blood cell count

34 A 54-year-old man has been prescribed a catechol-O-methyltransferase (COMT) inhibitor to treat Parkinson's disease. He is concerned about the reports of fatal liver toxicity associated with this drug.

Which one of the following medicines was most likely prescribed for this patient?

    ☐ **A**   cabergoline
    ☐ **B**   entacapone
    ☐ **C**   rasagiline
    ☐ **D**   selegine
    ☐ **E**   tolcapone

35 A 65-year-old female has suffered a minor stroke and has been admitted to hospital. Her records indicate a history of DVT, type 2 diabetes, hypertension and hypercholesterolaemia.
Which one of her following medicines should be discontinued?

    ☐ **A**   atorvastatin
    ☐ **B**   enoxaparin
    ☐ **C**   metformin
    ☐ **D**   ramipril
    ☐ **E**   sitagliptin

36 A 70-year-old male who is suffering from lung cancer is undergoing treatment with vincristine. He starts to feel a painful stinging sensation at the injection site and you suspect the drug is being extravasated.
Which one of the following factors is LEAST likely to increase the risk of extravasation?

    ☐ **A**   age
    ☐ **B**   concurrent administration of simvastatin
    ☐ **C**   lymphoedema
    ☐ **D**   obesity
    ☐ **E**   presence of peripheral neuropathy

37 A 27-year-old female presents with the following symptoms: weight loss, anxiety, tachycardia and insomnia.
Which one of the following medicines may be contributing to these symptoms?

    ☐ **A**   azithromycin 1g
    ☐ **B**   citalopram 20 mg
    ☐ **C**   levothyroxine 200 mcg
    ☐ **D**   *Microgynon 30*®
    ☐ **E**   propanolol 160 mg

38 A 28-year-old male presents at the pharmacy with a scaly rash on his left foot and has cracks in between his toes. Upon further questioning the patient tells you that the rash has lasted 3 weeks and complains of stinging, burning and itchiness.

Which one of the following counselling points is LEAST appropriate for this patient?

- [ ] **A** Use talcum powder to help prevent your feet from getting sweaty
- [ ] **B** Griseofulvin is first-line treatment for this condition
- [ ] **C** Wear protective shoes in public showers
- [ ] **D** Avoid use of topical hydrocortisone creams
- [ ] **E** Apply clotrimazole two to three times a day for at least 4 weeks

39 A 59-year-old female with type 2 diabetes presents at the pharmacy requesting treatment for a fungal toenail infection. You suspect she has onychomycosis and refer her to the podiatrist.
Which one of the following statements is correct with regards to onychomycosis?

- [ ] **A** Cure is not achieved in 5–10% of patients
- [ ] **B** It is rare in patients with diabetes
- [ ] **C** Nails will appear normal within 3 months
- [ ] **D** Relapse occurs in about 5–10 % of people
- [ ] **E** Without treatment the condition often spreads to multiple toenails

40 A 20-year-old male with ulcerative colitis is admitted into hospital after presenting with fresh blood in his stools and suffering from diarrhoea with more than 8 stools per day. He is dehydrated with dry mucus membranes and an elevated heart rate of 110 bpm. An abdominal X-ray comes back normal with no evidence of obstruction or dilatation and blood tests also show inflammatory markers are within target range.
Which one the following treatment options is most appropriate for this patient?

- [ ] **A** Administer 1 L 5% dextrose IV over 24 hours
- [ ] **B** Administer cefuroxime 1.5 g hourly
- [ ] **C** Administer hydrocortisone 100 mg QDS IV
- [ ] **D** Administer metronidazole 500 mg TDS IV
- [ ] **E** Administer two loperamide 2 mg capsules straightaway, followed by one 2 mg capsule after each loose stool

Extended matching questions

Akila Ahmed and Pratik Thakkar

In this section, for each numbered question, select the one lettered option that most closely corresponds to the answer. Within each group of questions each lettered option may be used once, more than once or not at all.

Adverse drug reactions

    A   agranulocytosis
    B   aplastic anaemia
    C   haemolytic anaemia
    D   megaloblastic anaemia
    E   neutropenia
    F   thrombocytopenia

For questions 1–3

For the patient's symptoms described below, select the most likely ADR from the list above. Each option may be used once, more than once, or not at all.

1   A 56-year-old man attended his GP and was initiated on co-beneldopa 50/12.5 mg for his Parkinson's disease. Four weeks later he comes back to the GP. He presents with shortness of breath, jaundice and his urine is dark in colour.

2   A 65-year-old women was admitted to the emergency department at her local hospital. On admission she had a temperature of 37°C. She presented with lethargy, shortness of breath and had felt generally unwell for several weeks. On examination she had a dry cough but not

chest pain. Her past medical history includes rheumatoid arthritis and she was prescribed azathioprine. Her other medication includes folic acid, lansoprazole and ferrous sulphate. Her full blood count was:

- white cell count 1.0 (4.0–11.0 × 10^9/L)
- neutrophils 0.5 (2.5–7.5 × 10^9/L)
- haemoglobin 8.5 (11.5–15.5 g/dL)

3   An 83-year-old woman was started on sodium valproate for partial seizures. Four weeks later she has noticed bruising on the arms and legs.

Electrolyte abnormalities

A   hypercalcaemia
B   hyperkalaemia
C   hypernatraemia
D   hypocalcaemia
E   hypokalaemia
F   hyponatraemia

For questions 4–6

For the patients described below, select the most likely drug-induced cause of the patient's symptoms from the list above. Each option may be used once, more than once, or not at all.

4   Mr Albedi, an 88-year-old man was admitted 5 days ago following a fall. On your ward round you reviewed his list of medication before admission and the results of blood tests done following admission. His drug history included the following:

- bisoprolol 5 mg OD
- ramipril 10 mg OD
- furosemide 20 mg OM
- simvastatin 20 mg ON
- warfarin as per INR

You have identified K^+ 6.6 mmol/L, heart rate 60 beats per minute with ECG changes (tall T waves).

5   A 77-year-old woman was admitted to the ED with symptoms of confusion, agitation, fatigue and dizziness. She had been to see her GP 1 month ago with symptoms of feeling low and she was commenced on citalopram 20 mg OD.

6 Mrs McGee was presented to the assessment unit with vomiting and diarrhoea. She was on digoxin 125 mcg OD.

Rivaroxaban (oral tablet)

A   Rivaroxaban 2.5 mg taken orally twice daily for 12 months
B   Rivaroxaban 10 mg taken orally once daily for 2 weeks
C   Rivaroxaban 10 mg taken orally once daily for 5 weeks
D   Rivaroxaban 15 mg taken orally once daily
E   Rivaroxaban 15 mg taken orally twice daily
F   Rivaroxaban 15 mg twice daily for the first three weeks followed by 20 mg once daily for 3 months
G   Rivaroxaban 20 mg taken orally once daily

For questions 7–10

For the patients described below, select the most appropriate regimen from the list above. The patients have no known drug allergies or contraindications to rivaroxaban. Each option may be used once, more than once or not at all.

7   A 76-year-old man is taking the following medicines:

- atorvastatin 40 mg once daily
- esomeprazole 40 mg once daily
- metformin 500 mg twice daily
- ramipril 5 mg once daily

He has a history of type 2 diabetes and had a transient ischaemic attack 2 years ago. He has just been diagnosed with atrial fibrillation and the cardiologist decides to commence him on rivaroxaban.
You may use the BNF monograph for rivaroxaban tablets and the SPC for rivaroxaban tablets to help you: https://www.medicines.org.uk/emc/product/6402/smpc

8   A 45-year-old woman weighs 70 kg and has a CrCl of 84 mL/min. She presents with dyspnoea and tachypnoea. Patient history shows that she was in hospital 1 month ago for gastric surgery. In the last 24 hours she has been feeling unwell. She is taking the following medicines:

- levothyroxine sodium 100 micrograms once daily
- paracetamol 1 g every 6 hours when required

The consultant diagnoses a PE and has requested rivaroxaban.
You may use the BNF monograph for rivaroxaban tablets and the SPC for rivaroxaban tablets to help you: https://www.medicines.org.uk/emc/product/6402/smpc

9   A 70-year-old man weighs 60 kg and has a past medical history: type 2 diabetes, DVT, congestive cardiac failure and hypertension. He has been admitted to hospital with moderate-severity community-acquired pneumonia and dehydration. He is currently on the following medication:

  - bisoprolol 3.75 mg once daily
  - bumetanide 1 mg once daily
  - doxycycline 100 mg twice daily for 7 days
  - glicalazide 80 mg once daily
  - perindopril 4 mg once daily
  - rivaroxaban 20 mg once daily

The rivoroxaban dose for venous thromboembolism (VTE) prophylaxis will need to be amended. He has a CrCl of 40 mL/min.

You may use the BNF monograph for rivaroxaban tablets and the SPC for rivaroxaban tablets to help you: https://www.medicines.org.uk/emc/product/6402/smpc

10   A 52-year-old man is taking the following medicines:

  - atorvastatin 40 mg once daily
  - aspirin 75 mg
  - ramipril 2.5 mg once daily
  - isosorbide mononitrate XL 60 mg OD
  - GTN spray as needed

He was admitted with chest pain and has just been diagnosed with non-ST segment elevation myocardial infarction with elevated cardiac enzymes. The cardiologist wishes to start the patient on rivaroxaban.

You may use the BNF monograph for rivaroxaban tablets and the SPC for rivaroxaban tablets to help you: https://www.medicines.org.uk/emc/product/6402/smpc

Adverse drug reactions

  A   aspirin
  B   clonazepam
  C   co-trimoxazole
  D   efavirenz
  E   phenytoin
  F   sumatriptan
  G   *Yasmin*® (drospirenone and oestrogen)
  H   zidovudine

For questions 11–13

For the patients described below, select the most appropriate answer from the list above. Each option may be used once, more than once or not at all. You may use the BNF section on acute porphyrias to help you.

11 A patient presents to A&E with acute porphyria symptoms and is being initiated on treatment for this. She has never been diagnosed with the disease previously. You review her medications she bought with her listed below:

- aspirin
- co-amoxiclav
- sumatriptan
- *Yasmin*® (drospirenone and oestrogen)

Which one is most likely needed to be stopped as a result of the suspected porphyria?

12 A patient with porphyria has presented with an epileptic seizure. Which anticonvulsant is appropriate to use without further complications?

13 This virology product would be deemed unsuitable for a patient who has been diagnosed with HIV.

Special populations

A amoxicillin
B carbimazole
C metformin
D omeprazole
E orlistat
F paracetamol
G ranitidine
H simvastatin

For questions 14–16

For the patients described below, select the most appropriate drug to be discontinued from the list above. Each option may be used once, more than once or not at all.

14 A 40-year-old woman weighing 95 kg with type 2 diabetes mellitus has recently tested positive for pregnancy. She is currently taking the following medication:

- simvastatin 20 mg OD

- omeprazole 20 mg OD
- paracetamol 1 g QDS
- metformin 1 g OD

15 An elderly patient presents to the clinic and visually has deteriorated since the last time you saw them. The patient has significantly lost muscle tone around his arms and legs and is unable to perform strenuous tasks properly.

16 A patient presents to the pharmacy asking for lozenges and paracetamol for a fever and sore throat. You refer them to the GP for an urgent clinical review.

Mechanism of action

A   aciclovir
B   adalimumab
C   avelumab
D   carbidopa
E   ganciclovir
F   rituximab
G   sodium cromoglicate
H   suxamethonium

For questions 17–20

For the mechanisms of action described below, select the most appropriate product from the list above. Each option may be used once, more than once or not at all.

17 A peripheral decarboxylase inhibitor molecule that is commonly combined with levodopa to reduce risk of side effects in other tissues.

18 A drug which metabolises the mast cell membrane, inhibiting vasoactive mediators.

19 A monoclonal antibody that binds to CD20 on B cells.

20 A drug that binds to the nicotinic acetylcholine receptor in skeletal muscles acting as a depolarising neuromuscular blocking agent.

Converting opioids

A   10 mg
B   20 mg
C   30 mg
D   40 mg
E   50 mg
F   60 mg
G   70 mg
H   80 mg

For questions 21–23

For the patients described below, select the most appropriate answer from the list above based on BNF guidelines. Each option may be used once, more than once or not at all.

21 A patient has been admitted to the ward and has been taking oral morphine at a dose of 40 mg OD. What is the equivalent IV dose of morphine to be prescribed?

22 A clinician asks you what the equivalent dose of codeine PO 100 mg/day is for oral morphine.

23 A patient needs to be prescribed maximum oral morphine PRN for his breakthrough pain. He is currently on 2 sachets of *MST Continus*® 30 mg a day.

Drug interactions

A   allopurinol
B   ceftriaxone
C   ciprofloxacin
D   co-amoxiclav
E   flucloxacillin
F   isosorbide mononitrate
G   simvastatin
H   spironolactone

For questions 24–27

For the patients described below, select the most appropriate drug from the list above. Each option may be used once, more than once or not at all.

24 A patient with brittle asthma who is on theophylline is started on an antibiotic for an ear infection. Shortly within a few days they present with severe palpitations.

25 A patient with erectile dysfunction is about to be initiated on sildenafil. Which of the above medications is likely to interact with sildenafil?

26 You are checking a patient's blood results and notice that their potassium levels are elevated. When inquiring the medication history, you discover that amongst the medications they are on, they are also taking potassium supplements.

27 A patient with a penicillin allergy was recently started on clarithromycin for community-acquired pneumonia. They presented to the GP a week later with complaints of widespread muscle pain. Which of the above medications should have been stopped when the antibiotic was started?

Asthma/COPD medications

A   beclometasone
B   budesonide/formoterol
C   fluticasone and salmeterol
D   oral prednisolone
E   salbutamol
F   salmeterol
G   theophylline
H   tiotropium

For questions 28–30

For the patients described below, select the most appropriate product to use from the list above. Each option may be used once, more than once or not at all.

28 Mr B, a 15-year-old male patient, comes in complaining of night time cough with a family history of eczema and allergies.

29 A patient with an infective exacerbation of COPD has been admitted to the hospital. Which medication would be appropriate to optimise their outcome?

30 This product is available as an inhalation powder to use via a breath-actuated inhaler and a soft mist inhaler via inhalation solution.

SECTION B

Ryan Hamilton

In this section, for each numbered question, select the one lettered option that most closely corresponds to the answer. Within each group of questions each lettered option may be used once, more than once or not at all.

Antibacterials

    A   amoxicillin
    B   clindamycin
    C   co-trimoxazole
    D   doxycycline
    E   erythromycin
    F   linezolid
    G   meropenem
    H   vancomycin

For questions 1–10

For the patients described below, select the single most likely antibacterial agent implicated from the list above. Each option may be used once, more than once, or not at all.

1   Mrs G has been admitted to your assessment clinic from her GP after she was found to have hyperkalaemia. When looking at her medical records you find that she has been taking spironolactone for her established liver impairment and has recently been prescribed a long-term course of an antibiotic intended to protect her against bacterial peritonitis.

2   Mr D suffers from epilepsy and takes *Epilim Chrono*® (sodium valproate M/R) 500 mg BD, which has controlled his condition for a number of years. He has recently been prescribed an antibiotic for a severe infection but has subsequently suffered from a seizure. You check his valproate levels and they come back as severely sub-therapeutic. You suspect his antibiotic treatment has caused this.

3   Mr R has been taking simvastatin 40 mg at night since having a myocardial infarction and subsequently being diagnosed with familial hypercholesterolaemia. He was recently diagnosed with a respiratory

tract infection, for which his GP prescribed an antibiotic. Towards the end of the course Mr R complains of muscle pains and cramps and you advise him to stop his atorvastatin whilst taking this antibiotic.

4   Mr K has been taking isotretinoin for severe acne and his GP has recently prescribed a course of an antibiotic to cover any bacterial involvement. Unfortunately, Mr K started complaining of severe headaches and visual disturbances. The neurology team at your hospital diagnose him with cranial hypertension and you suggest there has been an interaction between his antibiotic treatment and isotretinoin.

5   Mrs J has recently been admitted to your cardiac unit with palpitations caused by a prolonged QT interval. When you take her drug history you find she has been using domperidone for a number of years when required for nausea. However, she has recently been prescribed a course of antibiotics for a skin infection which caused her to feel sick so she has been taking her domperidone more often. You believe the additive side effects, and a possible interaction, between domperidone and this antibiotic have caused her prolonged QT interval.

6   Miss C has just been admitted to your emergency department with hyperthermia, altered mental state, muscle spasms and urinary retention. The medical team diagnose her as having possible serotonin syndrome and prescribe dantrolene to prevent muscle spasms and damage. When taking her drug history you find she takes fluoxetine 60 mg daily for depression and was recently prescribed an antibiotic for cellulitis. You believe this antibiotic therapy has interacted with the fluoxetine to precipitate the serotonin syndrome.

7   Mr W has been admitted to your ward with profuse diarrhoea but no vomiting. He feels unwell and feverish, and has a white cell count of 21.6×10^9/L and an albumin of 28 g/L. The medical team asks for your advice on an antibiotic as Mr W has been in hospital twice in the last 6 months and has had multiple courses of antibiotics for chest infections.

8   Neil is a 6-year-old boy who has been diagnosed with cellulitis caused by MRSA. The medical team are contemplating prescribing this antibiotic, but you warn them it can bind to developing bone and discolour teeth.

9   Mr J has recently been prescribed this antibiotic for the treatment of osteomyelitis secondary to his infected diabetic foot ulcer. He has been taking this antibiotic for 4 weeks and has attended the diabetic foot

clinic for review of his ulcer and blood tests. While his ulcer is healing well, the blood tests show that his white cell, red cell, and platelet counts have all dropped significantly and he is complaining of having flu-like symptoms. You believe it is due to the antibiotic that Mr J is taking.

10 Mrs O has been admitted to your emergency department with a painful and progressive rash. The dermatology team diagnose Mrs O with Stevens-Johnson syndrome and she is transferred to ITU for acute management. Whilst completing her medication history you find Mrs O does not usually take any medicines regularly or acutely, but was prescribed an antibiotic from her GP last week, which she was still taking up to admission. You believe this antibiotic may have caused her current condition.

Antihypertensives and diuretics

A amlodipine
B bendroflumethiazide
C candesartan
D furosemide
E labetalol
F metolazone
G ramipril
H spironolactone

For questions 11–15

For the patients described below, select the single most likely medication from the list above. Each option may be used once, more than once, or not at all.

11 Mr N suffers from hepatitis and cirrhosis, which has recently progressed to decompensated liver disease. This has resulted in the development of ascites within Mr N's abdomen. To reduce fluid accumulation, the gastroenterology team wants to prescribe this medicine for Mr N.

12 Mrs A is an 83-year-old woman who has been successfully treated for hypertension for the past 21 years with this medicine. She attends your hypertension clinic today and you find her average blood pressure, from three readings, to be 151/93 mmHg. Nothing has changed in her lifestyle but her recent blood tests show her eGFR is now only 26 mL/min and you believe her antihypertension medicine is no longer effective because of this.

13 Mrs D is a 71-year-old woman who comes into your pharmacy asking for advice about compression bandages for her legs. In the consultation room you find she has bilateral ankle oedema that has developed over the past 2 weeks. On further questioning you find she was started on a new medicine for her high blood pressure. You advise the patient to see her GP as you believe the ankle oedema to be secondary to this new medicine.

14 Mr P has been treated for hypertension for a number of years and is on a combination of medicines. When collecting his prescription you ask him how he is and he complains of developing "man boobs" that are sometimes "tender to touch". He has not gained weight and does not drink alcohol. You believe one of his hypertension medicines may be causing this gynaecomastia.

15 Miss M is 25 weeks pregnant and presents to the urgent care centre with nausea and dizziness. She is found to be hypertensive and the obstetrics team would like to start treatment to prevent damage to the foetus. This medicine is considered the first-line option for hypertension in pregnancy.

Diabetes

A dapagliflozin
B exenatide
C gliclazide
D insulin
E linagliptin
F liraglutide
G metformin
H pioglitazone
I tolbutamide

For questions 16–21

For the patients described below, select the single most likely agent from the list above. Each option may be used once, more than once, or not at all.

16 Mrs O has been diagnosed with diabetes and is struggling to tolerate the first-line agents. Her GP started her on a new treatment that has controlled her blood sugar much better, but she has experienced a number of thrush and UTI episodes since starting this medicine.

You contact her GP to discuss this as you think this medicine might have contributed to the increased incidence of infection.

17 Mr A is well known to your diabetes clinic but is struggling to reduce his HbA1c so you decide to prescribe an additional medicine. When checking his medical records you note that he has recently been referred to the urology clinic to investigate haematuria. You are concerned that bladder cancer needs to be ruled out before prescribing this medicine.

18 Mr B has been admitted to your ward with acute heart failure. When reviewing his medicines you suggest that his medical team withhold this antihyperglycaemic agent as he will be at increased risk of lactic acidosis because of this medicine.

19 Ms D has insulin-dependent diabetes mellitus and is currently on an intense insulin regimen that isn't controlling her blood sugar levels. She is overweight and her consultant believes she is developing insulin resistance. The consultant prescribes Ms D an oral agent that should increase insulin utilisation in the body, in turn helping her lose weight and reduce her insulin dose.

20 Mr U has type 2 diabetes and was taking a first-line agent for a number of years but now requires his treatment to be stepped up. When advising on which agent to add in to his therapy you specifically advise against the use of one drug because he was discharged from hospital 6 months ago after suffering a myocardial infarction, which has resulted in mild congestive heart failure.

21 Mr N is a 26-year-old man who weighs 307 kg. He does not have diabetes and has changed his diet to promote weight loss. He has been seen by a specialist in weight loss who has prescribed this medicine to drive further weight loss.

Epilepsy

A clobazam
B diazepam
C lamotrigine
D levetiracetam
E lorazepam
F phenobarbital
G phenytoin
H sodium valproate

For questions 22–26

For the patients described below, select the single most likely medication from the list above. Each option may be used once, more than once, or not at all.

22 Mr J is known to suffer from epilepsy and has been admitted to your hospital with status epilepticus, which has failed to resolve after administration of intravenous lorazepam. The medical team prescribe this anticonvulsant as a loading dose followed by an infusion. You ask the medical team to monitor the patient's ECG and blood pressure while the patient is receiving this medicine intravenously.

23 Mrs D has recently moved to your locality and brings in her prescription for this anticonvulsant medicine. You invite her into your consultation room for a conversation about her medicines. You find that she has not been warned about the risks of this medicine in women of childbearing age and advise her to see her GP as soon as possible for advice about pregnancy prevention, or alternative treatments.

24 Miss E has suffered from epilepsy since childhood and is generally seizure-free. However, she has been suffering from increased seizures and has been admitted to hospital having suffered two seizures this morning. In the emergency department she has a seizure lasting more than 5 minutes and the medical team administer this medicine intravenously to abate the convulsions.

25 Mr V has a complex seizure history and is currently on three different anticonvulsants to manage his condition. However, he is still having around one seizure per week and the neurology team add in another agent. This medicine is generally taken at bed time.

26 Miss C is 13 years old and has been taking this epilepsy medicine for a number of years which has kept her seizure free for the last 2 years. Miss C is concerned about her acne, which seems to be a lot worse than the other children at her school. She has tried a number of self-management options to no effect. You believe that her epilepsy medicine may be exacerbating her acne.

Electrolytes

A   ammonia (NH_3)
B   calcium carbonate ($CaCO^3$)
C   calcium gluconate ($CaC_{12}H_{22}O_{14}$)
D   chloride (Cl^-)
E   magnesium (Mg^+)
F   magnesium sulfate ($MgSO_4$)
G   potassium (K^+)
H   sodium (Na^+)
I   sodium bicarbonate ($NaHCO_3$)

> For questions 27–31
>
> For the patients described below, select the single most likely electrolyte from the list above. Each option may be used once, more than once, or not at all.

27   Mr X is a 68-year-old with a history of type 1 diabetes and chronic renal impairment. He has been admitted to hospital feeling generally unwell for the last week and is found to be acidotic (arterial blood gas pH = 7.28). The medical team ask your advice on what to give and you recommend an infusion of this electrolyte.

28   Mrs H is well known to your renal service and is currently awaiting a renal transplant. Her recent bloods show that she is suffering from hyperphosphatemia and this appears to have worsened over the past month. You recommend this electrolyte complex to reduce Mrs H's phosphate levels.

29   Miss D has been admitted to your hospital suffering from a severe acute exacerbation of asthma for which she is prescribed nebulised ipratropium 500 mcg QDS and nebulised salbutamol 5 mg PRN. While she has been responding to treatment clinically, her arterial blood gas shows depletion of this electrolyte so you recommend reducing the salbutamol to 2.5 mg PRN and giving intravenous supplements of this electrolyte.

30   Mr Y has been admitted to your hospital from his GP after blood tests showed his serum potassium was 6.6 mmol/L. In the emergency department he is given intravenous fluids and an ECG shows he has sinus tachycardia. Regardless, the acute medics would like to protect the myocardium and you suggest this electrolyte.

31 Mrs E is taking carbamazepine 100 mg twice daily, simvastatin 40 mg at night and mirtazapine 45 mg at night. She has been admitted to hospital with increasing confusion and drowsiness over the last week. The mirtazapine dose was increased from 30 mg at night about 2 weeks ago. Blood tests show her carbamazepine levels are in range and there are no signs of infection. However, her blood tests do show she has low levels of this electrolyte, which you think may be due to her medicines.

Evidence based medicine

A absolute risk reduction (ARR)
B confidence interval (CI)
C kappa score (κ)
D number needed to treat (NNT)
E odds ratio (OR)
F p value (p)
G relative risk reduction (RRR)
H standard deviation (SD)

For questions 32–36

For the statements described below, select the single most likely option from the list above. Each option may be used once, more than once, or not at all.

32 This value can describe the overall statistical significance of the difference between the intervention and the control groups in a clinical trial.

33 This is a measure of uncertainty. A wide range of numbers suggests an imprecise result and indicates that the results should be interpreted with caution regardless of statistical significance.

34 This is an estimate of the number of people who need to be given an intervention, or medicine, for one person to experience a positive outcome, or prevention of a negative outcome.

35 This is the reduction in risk as a proportion between two treatment groups or interventions. It can be considered as the percentage difference in risk between two study groups or interventions.

36 This number describes the difference of an event happening in one group compared to another group, given as an integer but represents a ratio.

Respiratory medicine

   A   aminophylline tablets 450 mg BD
   B   carbocisteine capsules 750 mg TDS
   C   ipratropium 500 mcg nebulised QDS
   D   prednisolone tablets 40 mg OD
   E   salbutamol 2.5 mg nebulised QDS
   F   salbutamol 5 mg nebulised QDS
   G   theophylline tablets 200 mg BD
   H   tiotropium 10 mcg dry power inhaler once daily

For questions 37–40

For the patients described below, select the single most likely respiratory medication from the list above. Each option may be used once, more than once, or not at all.

37 Miss Z is being treated for an acute exacerbation of asthma and while her blood gases show her condition is improving, her heart rate has increased and she appears to have developed a fine tremor in her hands. You believe this medicine might be responsible.

38 Mrs W has suffered from COPD for 14 years and has been stable on her inhalers for a number of years. However, the local GP surgery changed the device of one of her inhalers and she complains that she has been struggling to use this and you are concerned that she could be at risk of choking. You decide to counsel her on the use of this new device.

39 Mr V comes into your community pharmacy with a prescription for antibiotics and an inhaler to take for 7 days for community acquired pneumonia, which you are happy to dispense. However, he has also been prescribed a third medicine that you are not happy to dispense as you do not believe it will be effective within this time period. You decide to call the GP and discuss this third medicine.

40 Mrs T has COPD, which she has been struggling to manage and suffers from regular exacerbations. She presents to your urgent care centre with melaena and epigastric pain. After endoscopy she is diagnosed with a peptic ulcer and you recommend the medical team stop one of her COPD medicines.

SECTION C

Oksana Pyzik

In this section, for each numbered question, select the one lettered option that most closely corresponds to the answer. Within each group of questions each lettered option may be used once, more than once or not at all.

Antidepressants and anxiolytics

    A   amitriptyline
    B   buspirone
    C   citalopram
    D   nortriptyline
    E   sertraline
    F   trazodone
    G   venlafaxine
    H   zopiclone

For questions 1–5

For the patients described below, select the single most likely antidepressant and/or anxiolytic from the list above. Each option may be used once, more than once or not at all.

1   A 28-year-old male was treated with an antidepressant for 2 years, however, recently his depressive symptoms have worsened and anxiety heightened. His prescriber has suggested the following antidepressant of the serotonin and norepinephrine reuptake inhibitor class.

2   A 23-year-old female is suffering from anxiety. In addition to cognitive behavioural therapy (CBT), the prescriber has suggested medication starting at 5 mg two to three times a day for short term use.

3   A 54-year-old female with type 2 diabetes suffers from nerve pain and is prescribed an antidepressant which is unlicensed for neuropathic pain.

4   A 60-year-old male who suffers from depression has recently suffered a myocardial infarction and is switched to another antidepressant.

5   A 35-year-old female who has difficulties falling asleep with nocturnal awakening and early awakening is prescribed this medicine for 2–3 weeks.

Paediatric conditions

A   cradle cap
B   croup
C   hand, foot and mouth disease
D   impetigo
E   measles
F   meningitis
G   molluscum contagiosum
H   scarlet fever

For questions 6–10

For the scenarios described below, select the single most likely paediatric condition from the list above. Each option may be used once, more than once or not at all.

6   A 6-year-old boy presents with firm, smooth, umbilicated papules, about 2.5 mm in diameter under his armpit and behind his knees in clusters of 20 lesions in a row. The pink, waxy, dome-shaped growth is filled with a firm white substance and the child does not complain of any pain.

7   A 2-year-old presents with lesions that evolved rapidly into honey-coloured crusted plaques about 1.5 cm in diameter around the mouth and nose.

8   A 13-month-old child develops a barking cough and shortness of breath, and is subsequently treated with dexamethasone.

9   A 3-year-old child presents with a generalised petechial rash, fever, headache, photophobia and stiff neck, as well as Kernig's sign (pain and resistance on passive knee extension with hips fully flexed).

10   A 10-year-old child presents with pyrexia, conjunctivitis and a runny nose. One day later the child presents with small white spots inside the mouth and a harsh dry cough. Three days later a red blotchy rash developed on the head and neck and then spread down the body. The rash turned a brownish colour and then gradually faded over a few days.

Toxic adverse effects

A   cardiotoxicity
B   hepatotoxicity
C   nephrotoxicity
D   neurotoxicity
E   ototoxicity
F   photosensitivity
G   pulmonary toxicity
H   toxic epidermal necrolysis

For questions 11–17

For the drugs described below, select the single most likely toxic effect from the list above. Each option may be used once, more than once or not at all.

11 A 51-year-old male is prescribed cisplatin for lung cancer. Cisplatin may cause toxicity in up to 31% of patients treated with a single dose of cisplatin 50 mg/m^2, and is manifested by tinnitus.

12 A 42-year-old female has been prescribed doxorubicin for lymphoma. The oncologist requests various tests for monitoring because there is a risk of developing toxicity with doxorubicin. It is recommended not to exceed a lifetime maximum cumulative dose of 550 mg/m^2.

13 A 23-year-old patient has been prescribed bleomycin for Hodgkin's lymphoma. The earliest sign and symptom associated with dose and age-related toxicity caused by bleomycin are fine rales and dyspnoea respectively.

14 An 84-year-old male is admitted to A&E with severe bronchopneumonia and is treated with gentamicin. He is also taking ibuprofen and sulfasalazine for rheumatoid arthritis. He begins to display symptoms of oedema around his legs and ankles, chest pain, shortness of breath, fatigue, persistent nausea and confusion.

15 A 45-year-old-female has been initiated on amiodarone in hospital. She begins to develop widespread erythema and bullous detachment of the epidermis and mucous membranes, resulting in exfoliation. Amiodarone is immediately discontinued.

16 A 16-year-old male is prescribed isotretinoin for severe acne and is counselled to take protective measures.

17 A 47-year-old female requires treatment with amphotericin B for disseminated candidiasis. Serum creatinine, potassium and magnesium levels should be monitored regularly due to risk of this adverse effect.

Antiepileptics

   A   carbamazepine
   B   lamotrigine
   C   lorazepam
   D   phenytoin sodium
   E   primidone
   F   sodium valproate
   G   topirimate
   H   zonisamide

For questions 18–23

For the statements described below, select the single most likely antiepileptic from the list above. Each option may be used once, more than once or not at all.

18 A 68-year-old male develops trigeminal neuralgia and is prescribed the first-line treatment.

19 This medicine should be taken in a number of divided doses. Initially 100–200 mg once or twice a day, followed by a slow increase until the best response is obtained, often 800–1200 mg daily in divided doses. This medicine should be avoided in absence seizures as it may worsen the condition.

20 A 34-year-old female has a seizure that lasts 6 minutes and receives treatment intravenously. The patient is monitored for respiratory depression and hypotension.

21 Patients or their carers should be told how to recognise signs and symptoms of pancreatitis and advised to seek immediate medical attention if symptoms such as abdominal pain, nausea, or vomiting develop.

22 This medicine is contraindicated in patients with a personal or family history of severe hepatic dysfunction, especially drug-related, active liver disease and in patients with known urea cycle disorders.

23 This antiepileptic is highly teratogenic. Infants exposed to this drug in utero are at a high risk of serious developmental disorders (up to 30–40%) and congenital malformations (approximately 11% risk). It should not be used in female children or during pregnancy. Females of childbearing potential must not be prescribed this drug unless they are on the pregnancy prevention plan.

Vaccines

A   Bacillus Calmette-Guerin (BCG) vaccine
B   cholera vaccine
C   hepatitis A vaccine
D   hepatitis B vaccine
E   human papillomavirus vaccine
F   rabies vaccine
G   rotavirus vaccine
H   yellow fever vaccine

For questions 24–27

For the patients described below, select the single most likely vaccine from the list above. Each option may be used once, more than once or not at all.

24 A neonate at risk of tuberculosis receives a vaccine that is a live attenuate strain derived from *Mycobacterium bovis* which stimulates immunity to *M. tuberculosis*.

25 A 6-year-old male is prescribed an oral vaccine. You counsel the carer to dissolve effervescent sodium bicarbonate granules in a glassful of water or chlorinated water approximately 150 mL. Discard half, approximately 75 mL, of the solution, then add the vaccine suspension to make one dose and drink within 2 hours. Food, drink, and other oral medicines should be avoided for 1 hour before and after vaccination.

26 It is currently recommended in the UK that this vaccine is given to teenage girls as part of the standard immunisation schedule at school to prevent premalignant genital lesions, cervical and anal cancers and genital warts.

27 A 6-week-old infant is prescribed a live oral vaccine against gastroenteritis. The second dose is administered 4 weeks later.

Laboratory tests and other markers

A ALT
B Creatinine
C HbA1c
D HDL
E LDL
F MCV
G T4
H TSH

For questions 28–32

For the patients described below, select the single most likely laboratory
test or other marker from the list above. Each option may be used once,
more than once or not at all.

28 A 68-year-old male's test results indicate high levels of bad cholesterol
with 160–189 mg/dL.

Total cholesterol level	Category
Less than 200 mg/dL	Desirable
200–239 mg/dL	Borderline high
240 mg/dL and above	High

LDL (bad) cholesterol level	LDL cholesterol category
Less than 100 mg/dL	Optimal
100–129 mg/dL	Near optimal/above optimal
130–159 mg/dL	Borderline high
160–189 mg/dL	High
190 mg/dL and above	Very high

HDL (good) cholesterol level	HDL cholesterol category
60 mg/dL and higher	Considered protective against heart disease
40–59 mg/dL	The higher, the better
Less than 40 mg/dL	A major risk factor for heart disease

Source: https://medlineplus.gov/lab-tests/cholesterol-levels/

29 A 51-year-old male who may have Hashimoto's disease will have elevated levels of this marker through a compensatory mechanism.

30 A blood test is requested for a 40-year-old female with a suspected case of iron deficiency anaemia. The blood test reveals microcytic red blood cells.

31 A 51-year-old male with early signs of alcoholic liver cirrhosis has had a liver function test that has shown elevated levels of bilirubin and this marker.

32 A 72-year-old female is taking vancomycin and is dehydrated. You suspect she may be suffering from acute kidney injury.

Women's health

    A   abortion
    B   cervical cancer
    C   endometriosis
    D   fibromyalgia
    E   pelvic inflammatory disease
    F   polycystic ovary syndrome
    G   pre-eclampsia
    H   trichomoniasis

For questions 33–40

For the scenarios described below, select the single most likely condition or procedure from the list above. Each option may be used once, more than once or not at all.

33 A 23-year-old female is prescribed mifepristone to be taken as a single 600 mg (i.e. 3 tablets of 200 mg each) oral dose, followed by misoprostol 400 µg orally, 36 to 48 hours later.

34 A 44-year-old female complains of severe dysmenorrhea, menorrhagia, menometrorrhagia, fatigue, diarrhoea, constipation and bloating as well as pain during and after intercourse. Progestin therapy has failed and the GP has recommended a surgical intervention – hysterectomy and removal of both ovaries.

35 1 in 10 women of reproductive age in the UK suffer from this condition and it is linked to infertility. Although the exact cause of this condition is not certain, possible explanations include retrograde menstruation, transformation of peritoneal cells and embryonic cell transformation.

36 A 26-year-old female is 36 weeks pregnant and presents with epigastric pain and new onset of hypertension with a reading of 159/109 mmHg. Upon admission into hospital, a blood test is taken which shows elevated levels of protein in the urine (0.35 g of protein in a 24-hour urine collection).

37 A 27-year-old female complains of irregular periods, weight gain, hirsutism, mood swings, sleep apnoea, and acne. An ultrasound reveals an increased ovarian volume and 12 peripheral follicles.

38 An 18-year-old female presents with abnormal greenish vaginal discharge characterised by a pungent odour.

39 A 19-year-old female was fitted with an intrauterine device 2 weeks ago. She presents with symptoms of lower abdominal pain, mucopurulent cervical discharge, pyrexia and painful and frequent urination. The GP identifies uterine tenderness and adnexal tenderness. She has a history of previous chlamydia infections.

40 A 50-year-old woman is married with six children. She smokes 20 cigarettes a day and drinks on social occasions. She reports chronic urinary frequency and vaginal spotting after intercourse which she thinks is related to vaginal dryness after menopause. She has not had a routine check-up with her GP in over 15 years. You refer her for a routine screening test.

SECTION D

Sadia Qayyum and Sonia Kauser

In this section, for each numbered question, select the one lettered option that most closely corresponds to the answer. Within each group of questions each lettered option may be used once, more than once or not at all.

Minor ailments

    A   allergic conjunctivitis
    B   bacterial conjunctivitis
    C   headlice
    D   mouth ulcers
    E   oral thrush
    F   scabies
    G   verrucas
    H   warts

For questions 1–5

For the scenarios described below, select the most likely condition the patient is suffering from, from the list above. Each option may be used once, more than once or not at all.

1   A 22-year-old patient presents to you in the pharmacy suffering from a painful and gritty left eye. The symptoms started 2 days ago and she complains that she woke up this morning and her eye was full of a sticky discharge.

2   A mother asks you about her 12-year-old son who is complaining of an itchy scalp with some white dots attached to the hair close to the scalp.

3   A 45-year-old smoker who is complaining of four or five small painful lesions in his mouth. The lesions are white in the centre with a red outer edge. They are spread over the inside of his lips, cheeks and under the tongue.

4   A 6-month-old baby, whose mother is concerned about a thick white substance affecting the mouth, covering the baby's tongue and inside the cheeks.

5   A 17-year-old swimmer complaining of a sore area on the bottom of his foot. The sore is not weeping or bleeding but looks like there are black dots in the centre of it.

Legislation

A   72 hours
B   7 days
C   14 days
D   28 days
E   30 days
F   6 months
G   12 months
H   36 months

For questions 6–10

For the statements listed below, select the most likely time period from the list above. Each option can be used once, more than once or not at all.

6   The length of validity of a controlled drug prescription from the appropriate date.

7   Maximum length of time it is recommended to prescribe a controlled drug on a single prescription.

8   Maximum length of time an emergency supply can cover for prescription-only medicines.

9   Maximum length of time a prescriber has to provide a prescription following their request for an emergency supply for a patient.

10 Length of validity of a private prescription from the appropriate date.

Drug reactions

A   hyperglycaemia
B   hyperkalaemia
C   hypernatraemia
D   hypertension
E   hypoglycaemia
F   hypokalaemia
G   hyponatraemia
H   hypotension

For questions 11–15

For the patients described below, select the most likely adverse drug reaction from the list above. Each option can be used once, more than once or not used at all.

11 An elderly patient, aged 83, is admitted into an elderly medical admissions ward due to confusion and a fall. Her repeat prescription medication includes lansoprazole, codeine and furosemide.

12 Mrs GT, aged 56, presents to A&E with nausea and vomiting, fast and deep breathing and sleepiness. Her medication includes aspirin, metformin, empagliflozin, clopidogrel and pantoprazole.

13 Mrs AF, aged 59, presents with a recent onset of increased fatigue, weakness and tiredness. Her current medication includes warfarin, digoxin, furosemide, adcal and alendronic acid.

14 Mr FN, aged 80, is admitted into a medical admissions ward due to sweating and feeling dizzy. This has been ongoing for the past month. His medication includes metformin, gliclazide, codeine, ramipril, aspirin and bisoprolol.

15 Mr HB, aged 52, complains of a headache but has no other symptoms. He is attending for a routine review of his medication at the pharmacy. His current medication includes ramipril, amlodipine, clopidogrel, naproxen and paracetamol.

Calculation questions

SECTION A

Ryan Hamilton

Questions 1 and 2 concern Mrs R, who comes to see you about losing weight and would like to try orlistat. During the consultation you take some weights and measurements and find that Mrs R is 4 feet 11 inches tall and weighs 13 stones and 1 pound.

You may use the Approximate Conversions and Units page in the BNF to support your calculations.

1   What is Mrs R's body mass index (kg/m^2) expressed as a whole number?

2   How much weight (kg) does Mrs R need to lose to reach a healthy BMI of 24 kg/m^2? Give your answer to one decimal place.

3   Mr H is on your acute medical unit with suspected venous-catheter infection and the medical team would like to prescribe vancomycin. You look at Mr H's admission notes and discern the following information:

   - Age: 63 years old
   - Height: 1.8 m
   - Weight: 83 kg
   - BP: 150/95 mmHg
   - Serum potassium: 5.0 mmol/L
   - Serum creatinine: 2.26 mg/dL
   - Urea: 7.2 mmol/L

   What is Mr H's estimated creatinine clearance rate (mL/min)? Give your answer to one decimal place.

   You may use the SPC for IV vancomycin to help you: https://www.medicines.org.uk/emc/product/649/smpc

4   You are visiting a nursing home to undertake medicines reviews for the patients when you are approached by one of the medics. His patient Mrs B is currently taking *Zomorph*® (morphine sulfate M/R) capsules 60 mg twice daily. However, she is starting to experience regular breakthrough pain and rescue doses of *Oramorph*® (morphine sulfate 10 mg/5 mL) at one tenth of her total daily *Zomorph*® dose are not controlling the pain sufficiently. You mutually agree to increase the rescue dose of *Oramorph*® to one sixth of her total daily *Zomorph*® dose.
What would the dose (mg) be? Give your answer as a whole number.

5   Mr A has been admitted to your neurology ward and has had a nasogastric tube fitted. Upon taking his medication history you note he was taking phenytoin sodium capsules 150 mg twice daily to control his epilepsy. The medical team have prescribed phenytoin liquid, which you know is not bioequivalent.
How many millilitres of phenytoin suspension should Mr A receive for each dose?
You may use the SPC for phenytoin oral solution to help you: https://www.medicines.org.uk/emc/product/2257/smpc

6   Miss Y is going travelling and her GP calls you to discuss malaria prophylaxis as she will be visiting Nigeria. Miss Y will arrive in Abuja where she will stay for 1 week, before heading to visit family in a rural town for 2 weeks, then returning to the UK. You confirm that it will be unlikely for Miss Y to avoid exposure to the sun so you suggest that the GP prescribes *Malarone*® (atovaquone with proguanil hydrochloride) tablets once daily.
What is the minimum number of *Malarone*® tablets that should be prescribed for Miss Y?
You may use the Malaria, prophylaxis section of the BNF to help you with this question.

7   Mrs U is 26 weeks pregnant and suffers from iron-deficiency anaemia. A trial with oral ferrous sulphate failed to produce a significant response and the medical team now want to trial Mrs U on intravenous *Venofer*® (iron sucrose). You look in Mrs U's notes and find the following information:

- Age: 34 years old
- Height: 5′ 5″
- Weight before pregnancy: 58 kg
- Gestation: 26 weeks

- Iron: 5.3 micromol/L
- Haemoglobin: 9.0 g/dL
- BP: 130/80 mmHg

The consultant would like to aim for a haemoglobin level of 14 g/dL in Mrs U.

What is the total dose of iron (mg) this patient needs? Give your answer to the nearest 10 milligrams.

Total iron dose (mg)

= body weight (kg)

$\times$ {[target Hb (g/dL) − actual Hb (g/dL)] $\times$ 2.4} + χ

where χ is the milligrams of iron needed to replenish iron stores. $\chi = 500$ mg (or 15 mg/kg in patients weighing less than 35 kg).

8 Mr G has been admitted to your emergency department with suspected digoxin toxicity. After taking blood tests his serum digoxin level is found to be 3.7 micrograms/L and the medical team want to initiate *DigiFab*®. Mr G was weighed on admission as 69 kg.

No. DigiFab vials required

$$= \frac{[\text{patient weight (kg)} \times \text{digoxin level (micrograms/L)}]}{100}$$

How many whole vials of *DigiFab*® do you need to supply to adequately treat Mr G?

Questions 9 and 10 concern Bobby, a 12 year-old boy on your paediatric medical ward who has recently been receiving 10 mg methylprednisolone intravenously four times a day for severe inflammation. The medical team would like to transfer Bobby onto once daily oral prednisolone.

You may use the Glucocorticoid therapy, Glucocorticoid and mineralocorticoid activity section of the BNFC to help you with this question.

9 What dose (mg) should initially be prescribed? Give your answer to the nearest whole number.

10 On discharge the medical team would like to discharge Bobby on another two weeks of oral prednisolone 40 mg OD, until he is reviewed in clinic. How many prednisolone 5 mg tablets do you need to supply for Bobby on discharge?

11 You are working in a hospital aseptic unit and you are asked to produce a batch of 0.9% sodium chloride 1000 mL intravenous infusion bags, each containing 40 mmol of potassium.
How many millilitres of concentrated potassium chloride 15% w/v need to be added to each infusion bag? Give your answer to two decimal places.
Atomic weight of potassium = 39.0; atomic weight of chlorine = 35.5

12 You have received an order for 15 g of hydrocortisone cream 2%. Your pharmacy only has the 1% and 2.5% formulations available.
How much of the 1% cream (g) do you need to use in order to make the required product? Give your answer to the nearest whole number.

13 What weight (mg) of salicylic acid powder must you add to 50 g of 2% (w/w) salicylic acid cream to produce a cream of 5% (w/w)? Give your answer to the nearest whole number.

14 Mrs B comes into your pharmacy with a prescription for her 12 year old daughter who has been prescribed flucloxacillin 125 mg/5 ml suspension at a dose of 125 mg QDS for 7 days.
Given that when a 100 mL bottle of the suspension is made up it has an expiry date of 7 days, how many bottles should you supply? Give your answer to the nearest whole number.

15 Mrs F, who weighs 63.2 kg, requires an intravenous infusion of dopamine hydrochloride which has been prescribed at a rate of 3 micrograms/kg/minute. The nurses have pre-made infusion bags of 160 mg dopamine in 100 mL of glucose 5%.
Calculate the rate (mL/hour) at which the infusion pump should be set to. Give your answer to one decimal place.

16 Mr M is one of your septic arthritis patients and presents you with a prescription for IV flucloxacillin 2 g QDS to be administered through the local OPAT (outpatient parenteral antibacterial therapy) scheme. Each flucloxacillin 1 g vial is reconstituted in 20 mL water for injections, given over 30 minutes.
How many 10 mL water for injection ampoules should be supplied to cover the 5-week course? Give your answer to the nearest whole number.

17 Mr Z has been diagnosed with an acute flare of ulcerative colitis and has been prescribed prednisolone. You are given his prescription and note he has been placed on a weaning dose of prednisolone. Mr Z is required to take a high dose of prednisolone 50 mg OD for 14 days then wean by 5 mg every week until zero.

How many 5 mg prednisolone tablets should you supply to ensure Mr Z can complete the course? Give your answer to the nearest whole number.

18 Mrs J has HIV and is required to take co-trimoxazole for prophylaxis against *Pneumocystis jirovecii* (*Pneumocystis carinii*) infection at a dose of 960 mg each morning and evening on Mondays, Wednesdays and Fridays. Your pharmacy stocks the 480 mg strength of co-trimoxazole. How many 480 mg co-trimoxazole tablets are required to cover a 6-month (28-week) period? Give your answer to the nearest whole number.

19 Mr V has been newly diagnosed with pulmonary tuberculosis and his medical team are going to start the standard quadruple drug therapy as per national guidance. On the ward round you note that Mr V is obese and ask the nursing team to weigh the patient and get a height. After the ward round, his height is recorded as 5′ 9″ and he weighs 146 kg. You consult the TB drug monographs website (www.tbdrugmonographs .co.uk) and find the following information for ethambutol.
What daily dose should the medical team prescribe for Mr V? Give your answer to the nearest whole number.

ETHAMBUTOL DOSAGE

<u>Adults:</u> 15 mg/kg once daily (oral); or for DOT supervised regimen: 30 mg/kg three times per week. (Round the dose up or down to the closest whole number of tablets).

Obesity: Use ideal body weight plus 40% of the excess weight in markedly obese patients.

Male ideal body weight (kg) = 50 + (2.3 × height in inch above 5 foot)

Female ideal body weight (kg)

$$= 45.5 + (2.3 × \text{height in inch above 5 foot})$$

<u>Children (1 month to 18 years):</u> 20 mg/kg once daily (oral); or for DOT supervised regimen: 30 mg/kg three times per week. (Doses should be rounded down to facilitate administration of suitable volumes of liquid or an appropriate strength of tablet).

PREPARATIONS

Oral: 100 mg, 400 mg tablets

20 Mr R is suffering from heart failure and his consultant wants to trial a maintenance dose of intravenous digoxin, aiming for a serum digoxin concentration of 2.0 micrograms/L (acceptable range 1.5–2.0 micrograms/L).

Estimate the daily dose that Mr R should be prescribed. Give your answer to the nearest 5 mcg.

You take the following information from his notes:

Weight: 73 kg	**Height:** 5′ 10″	**Age:** 68 years old
HR: 93 bpm	**BP:** 130/80	**Temp:** 37°C
Creatinine: 115 μmol/L	**K⁺:** 3.7 mmol/L	**Urea:** 4.1 mmol/L
Creatinine clearance = 48.52 mL/min		

$$C_{pss} = \frac{(F \times D)}{(DigCl \times t)}$$

Non-heart failure DigCl (L/hr) = [0.06 × creatinine clearance (mL/min)]
+ [0.05 × IBW (kg)]

Heart failure DigCl (L/hr) = [0.053 × creatinine clearance (mL/min)]
+ [0.02 × IBW (kg)]

Male IBW = 50 kg + 2.3 kg for every inch over 5 ft

Female IBW = 45.5 kg + 2.3 kg for every inch over 5 ft

21 Mrs C has been admitted to your stroke unit after suffering from an ischaemic stroke. You complete her drug history and find that she was taking one 20 mg citalopram tablet and one 10 mg citalopram tablet each morning for depression. As her swallow is compromised you decide to convert her medicines to liquids.

What is the minimum volume of citalopram oral drops that needs to be supplied to provide 28 days' treatment? Give your answer in millilitres (mL) to the nearest whole millilitre.

You may use the SPC for citalopram oral drops to help you: https://www.medicines.org.uk/emc/product/1392/smpc

22 You are a pharmacist working for a pharmaceutical company and are developing a new tablet which utilises a film coating technique. The current set up can coat 1200 tablets per hour and each tablet is covered by an average of 6 mcg of coating mixture. Traditionally, a 5% excess in coating mixture is made up to ensure sufficient supply for the whole process.

What is the minimum amount of coating mixture that is needed to complete a six-hour production? Give your answer to two decimal places.

23 You have received a prescription for Mrs Q, an 86-year-old woman, who is receiving end-of-life care and is developing swallowing problems. Her palliative team has written a prescription for five one-gram suppositories containing morphine sulfate 5 mg, which you make up extemporaneously. You find the displacement value of morphine sulfate is 1.6 and work out a formula.
How much *Witepsol®* in grams would you need to make the necessary suppositories, including one extra to allow for an excess? Give your answer to two decimal places.

24 Mr E is a 76-year-old patient on your gastroenterology unit who has undergone complex surgery. Before admission he was taking one co-beneldopa 12.5/50 mg capsule and one pramipexole 350 microgram tablet three times a day and one co-beneldopa 25/100 mg M/R capsule at night for Parkinson's disease. The medical team are worried about these medicines being omitted, as it will impede recovery, so they ask you to convert him to a rotigotine patch.
What strength of rotigotine patch (mg/24 hours) should Mr E be prescribed?
You may use the Emergency Management of Patient's With Parkinson's guide from Parkinson's UK to help you: https://www.parkinsons.org.uk/sites/default/files/2017-12/pk0135_emergencymanagement.pdf

25 Mrs A is one of your regular warfarin patients who has just attended the anticoagulation clinic. Upon inspecting her warfarin book you note she is now prescribed warfarin 1 mg and 2 mg on alternate days.
Assuming her next dose will be 2 mg, how many warfarin 1 mg tablets do you need to supply Mrs A to last her 4 weeks? Give your answer to the nearest whole number.

26 Mr N is due to commence a course of fludarabine and his oncologist would like to dose him at 40 mg/m^2. You look at Mr N's notes and find that he is 1.62 m tall and weighs 82 kg.
Calculate the dose of fludarabine that should be prescribed to the nearest milligram.

$$BSA\ (m^2) = \sqrt{([height\ (cm) \times weight\ (kg)] \div 3600)}$$

27 You are working within the antimicrobial pharmacist team in your hospital and are looking at making cost savings across the regularly used drugs. The current standard meropenem regimen is 1 g TDS for 5 days and you decide to determine what cost savings can be achieved by switching patients from meropenem 1 g TDS for 5 days to meropenem

500 mg QDS for 5 days. Your purchasing department obtains packs of 10 meropenem 500 mg vials at a cost of £76.90 and packs of 10 meropenem 1 g vials at a cost of £153.50.

Calculate the expected cost saving per 100 patients by undertaking this switch. Give your answer to the nearest whole pound sterling (£).

28 You are working in a specialist IMP manufacturing unit and are asked about making an intrathecal infusion of 2.5% amphotericin B soluble. You know the product will need to be isotonic with the CSF, of which you find the average freezing point to be -0.5770°C. From your research you learn you may need to add sodium chloride to the formulation to make it isotonic. You find the freezing point depression value of a 1% sodium chloride solution to be 0.5760°C and the freezing point depression value of a 1% solution of soluble amphotericin to be 0.1242°C.

Calculate how much sodium chloride must be included in 5 mL of product to ensure it is isotonic. Give your answer to two decimal places.

$$W = \frac{f - a}{b}$$

W is the amount (% w/v) of adjusting compound to be added
f is the freezing point depression of the target body fluid
a is the freezing point depression of the drug solution(s)
b is the freezing-point depression of a 1% solution of adjusting compound

29 Mrs I has come to your Healthy Living Pharmacy for advice and support for alcohol consumption. You discuss what she drinks on an average week and find that she will drink a bottle (750 mL) of white wine every night. Upon further questioning you find that it is "standard" white wine which is approximately 11% ABV.

Estimate how many units of alcohol Mrs I drinks each week. Give your answer to the nearest whole unit.

30 Mr K has been advised to use 5 mL of hydrogen peroxide solution 10 vols, diluted in two parts of water, as a mouthwash, twice a day for the next 2 weeks. In your pharmacy you only stock the strong hydrogen peroxide solution 9% (30 vols) BP.

What is the minimum quantity (mL) of the hydrogen peroxide solution 9% (30 vols) that needs to be supplied to Mr K? Give your answer to the nearest whole millilitre.

SECTION B

Oksana Pyzik

1 A 21-year-old male who is allergic to peanuts accidentally ingests peanut butter. He is given an intramuscular injection of 0.5 mg of adrenaline 1 in 1000.
What volume of solution was he given? Give your answer to one decimal place.

2 As a medicines information pharmacist you are required to calculate the 'number needed to treat' (NNT) value for an injectable drug, erenumab, to treat chronic migraine. The drug is thought to disable a protein known as calcitonin gene-related peptide. Previous research found this protein may play a part in migraine symptoms. A meta-analysis from randomised double-blind clinical trials conducted over several months and a review of these trials demonstrated the following results:

- With erenumab 636/955 (67%) patients had the number of migraine attacks reduced by at least half
- With placebo 291/955 (30%) had the same outcome

Calculate the NNT value. Give your answer to the nearest whole number.

Formulae:

Experimental event rate (EER)
Control event rate (CER)
Absolute risk reduction (ARR) = EER − CER
Relative risk = EER/CER
Relative risk reduction (RRR) = ARR/CER
Number needed to treat (NNT) = 1/ARR

3 A 53-year-old male patient weighing 90 kg is given 4 mL of 50 mg in 5 mL solution by slow IV injection.
How much drug has he received? Give your answer to the nearest whole number.

4 A 24-year-old female with type 1 diabetes is 32 weeks pregnant and her blood pressure is 149/100 mmHg. She has 0.36 g of protein in a 24-hour urine collection and is diagnosed with pre-eclampsia. How much sodium chloride (NaCl) 0.9% would you need to add to a 2 mL ampoule of hydralazine 20 mg/2 mL to make a 1 mg/1 mL dilution? Give your answer to the nearest whole number.

5   A 50-year-old female weighing 68 kg is administered zopiclone 7.5 mg
for the treatment of insomnia. Immediately after administration the
plasma level of zopiclone is measured at 75 mcg/mL.
If the half-life of zopiclone is 5 hours, what is the plasma concentration
in mcg/mL after 1200 min? Give your answer to two decimal places.

6   A 16-year-old girl weighing 50 kg requires a 2 mg/kg slow IV bolus of
an antibiotic. The ampoule contains 50 mg in 2 mL.
What volume of solution is required? Give your answer to the nearest
whole number.

7   You are responsible for the budget of a clinic and suggest switching
from *FreeStyle*® blood glucose strips to *GlucoRx*® glucose strips to
create cost savings. There are currently 100 patients in the clinic who
receive 12 boxes of *FreeStyle*® strips each year.
How much can the clinic save each year by changing 100 patients to *GlucoRx*® strips? Give your answer to the nearest whole pound sterling (£).

8   A 28-year-old male has suffered severe injuries in a car accident and
requires treatment with morphine sulphate. While in hospital, his ability
to swallow medicines begins to deteriorate and thus an equivalent
injectable dose must be prepared.

60 mg morphine sulphate BD
Bioavailability of tablets = 0.3
IV injection = 1% (w/v)

Morphine sulphate is available as a 0.2% w/v solution for infusion.
Using the above information, how many mLs of this solution should
be recommended for each 24-hour interval? Give your answer to the
nearest whole millimetre.

9   A 59-year-old woman weighing 70 kg presents in the hospital with a
swollen right calf. Investigations reveal the following:

- D-dimer – positive
- Well's score – 6
- Serum creatinine – 66 µmol/L

Treatment with enoxaparin (LMW heparin) is initiated at a dose of 1.5
mg/kg or 150 units/kg.
What dose of enoxaparin in units do you give? Give your answer to the
nearest whole number.

10   A 5-year-old boy weighing 20 kg is prescribed ibuprofen 100 mg/5 mL
oral suspension for post-immunisation fever. You counsel the parent to

give 2.5 mL followed by one further dose of 2.5 mL six hours later. You advise that it is not recommended to give more than two doses in 24 hours.

In total, how much ibuprofen has been administered in mg? Give your answer to the nearest whole number.

11 A 9-year-old boy weighing 40 kg is prescribed rifampicin syrup 20 mg/kg/day for 5 days only. The maximum dose is 800 mg and the syrup is available at a concentration of 100 mg/5 mL.

What volume of rifampicin should be provided to cover this supply? Give your answer to the nearest whole number.

12 A 6-month-old infant weighing 8 kg is prescribed folic acid 500 mcg/kg/day. The folic acid syrup you have in stock contains 50 mg of folic acid per 100 mL.

What volume of folic acid syrup in mL should be given for a 28-day supply? Give your answer to the nearest whole number.

13 A 64-year-old male requires enteral feeding following gastrointestinal cancer surgery. He requires 2000 kcal per day and has been prescribed *Fresubin*® 1800 Complete which contains 180 kcal per 100 mL. Timing of feeding is very important and should occur at night for 10 hours.

Calculate the rate at which enteral feeding should be administered in mL/hour. Give your answer to the nearest whole millilitre per hour.

14 A 54-year-old woman presents a prescription for prednisolone tablets 5 mg. She has been prescribed a reducing dose after taking the prednisolone for the next 8 weeks to suppress an allergic disorder. Her initial dose of 60 mg daily is to be taken for another 10 days. At the end of the 10 days she is to reduce her daily dose by 5 mg once each week until the course is finished. You have in stock 147 tablets, and agree to supply her with 112 tablets to allow you to keep some for any further patients this afternoon. You will then owe her the rest, which you should have in stock tomorrow.

How many tablets will you owe the patient when she returns tomorrow? Give your answer to the nearest whole number.

15 An injection solution of botulinum toxin type B contains 2,000 units/ 0.5 mL of active ingredient. A hospital manufacturing unit is creating batches of 2 mL injection solution in ampoules to supply to local hospitals. Each batch size is 10 ampoules plus an extra 15% for QC batch testing.

How many units of botulinum toxin are needed to prepare two batches worth? Give your answer to the nearest whole number.

16 You conduct a review of patients with asthma who may be suitable for a dose reduction and highlight 12 patients on *Seretide*® 250 Evohaler who may be stepped down to *Seretide*® 125 Evohaler, and 7 patients who are on *Symbicort*® 400/12 Turbohaler who may be stepped down to *Symbicort*® 200/6 Turbohaler.

Inhaler	Cost
Seretide® 250 Evohaler (120 doses)	£59.48
Seretide® 125 Evohaler (120 doses)	£35.00
Symbicort® 400/12 Turbohaler (60 doses)	£38.00
Symbicort® 200/6 Turbohaler (120 doses)	£38.00

Considering there are 4 months left within the financial year, the surgery business manager asks you what the forecasted savings would be if all the patients were successfully stepped down.

Assume all *Seretide*® patients are using TWO puffs twice a day and all the *Symbicort*® patients are using ONE inhalation twice a day.

Counting 30 days as one month, what is the total saving for the practice over the next 4 months? Give your answer to the nearest whole pound sterling (£).

17 You are working for a pharmaceutical company where you are required to calculate the weight of potassium chloride in large quantities of solution before it is prepared.

How many grams of potassium chloride are needed to prepare 5 L of a solution containing 16 mmol of potassium ions per 20 mL? Give your answer to the nearest whole number.

Atomic weight of potassium = 39; atomic weight of chlorine = 35.5

18 A 68-year-old woman is currently on a heparin infusion to aid in the maintenance of catheter patency. It's 5pm and during your ward round you notice her pump is beeping and showing an occlusion, and you alert the nurse who presses the 'stop' button. The junior doctor arrives for his ward round and asks you how much heparin the patient has had so far today.

The last rate set on the pump was 1.75 mL/hour and it has not altered since it was set up at 8am this morning. Her prescription reads 20,000 units in 50 mL sodium chloride 0.9%.

How many units of heparin has the patient received so far? Give your answer to the nearest whole number.

19 A 73-year-old female suffers from tachycardia and has been taking three 62.5 mcg digoxin tablets every morning. Her symptoms have suddenly

worsened and she has been admitted to hospital. The prescriber asks the pharmacy team to prepare IV digoxin at the same dose as her oral regimen. She weighs 70 kg, height is 5′ 8″, and her serum creatinine is 90 μmol/L.

Estimate her serum concentration as a result of the IV digoxin. Give your answer to one decimal place.

$$\text{CrCl (mL/min)} = \frac{(140 - \text{age [years]}) \times \text{weight (kg)} \times F}{\text{SeCr (micromol/litre)}}$$

where F is 1.23 for males and 1.04 for females.

$$C_{pss} = \frac{(F \times D)}{(\text{DigCl} \times t)}$$

Non heart failure DigCl (L/hr)

$= (0.06 \times \text{Creatinine Clearance (mL/min)}) + (0.05 \times \text{IBW (kg)})$

20 You are preparing a batch of menthol suppositories using theobroma oil as a base.

Given that the displacement value for menthol is 0.6, what weight of theobroma oil base is required to prepare 40 suppositories each weighing 1.55 g and each containing 75 mg of menthol? Give your answer to one decimal place.

SECTION C

Sadia Qayyum

1   A 36-year-old patient weighing 71 kg has been prescribed *Oramorph*®
    concentrate oral solution 100 mg/5 mL. The prescribed dose is 90
    mg when required up to a maximum of four times a day for break-
    through pain.
    Calculate the volume in mL required for each dose for breakthrough
    pain. Give your answer to one decimal place.

2   A doctor prescribes 500 mg amoxicillin capsules with directions for the
    patient to take ONE capsule THREE times a day for FIVE days.
    Calculate, in grams, the total weight of amoxicillin taken by the patient
    by the end of the course. Give your answer to one decimal place.

3   A 52-year-old woman has been prescribed co-codamol 30/500 mg
    soluble tablets. The dose she has been taking is TWO tablets FOUR
    times a day. Each tablet contains 388 mg of sodium. The recommended
    daily allowance (RDA) of salt for an adult is 6 g (equivalent to 2.4 g
    sodium) per day.
    What percentage of this patient's recommended daily sodium allowance
    is contained in a total daily dose of co-codamol 30/500 mg soluble
    tablets? Give your answer to one decimal place.

4   A 59-year-old female patient who weighs 69 kg, has been admitted onto
    your ward. Her latest serum creatinine level is 275 micromol/L. She has
    been prescribed a new medication, drug Y, which is mostly excreted
    through the kidneys. The dose of drug Y needs to be adjusted depending
    on the patient's renal function, calculated using the Cockcroft-Gault
    formula and applying as follows:

Creatinine clearance (mL/min)	Dosage
<10	5 mg/kg every 12 hours
10–20	10 mg/kg every 12 hours
21–35	15 mg/kg every 12 hours
35–50	15 mg/kg every 8 hours
>50	25 mg/kg every 8 hours

What dose of drug Y would you recommend to be taken over a 24-hour
period? Give your answer in grams to two decimal places.

Cockcroft-Gault formula:

$$\text{CrCl (mL/min)} = \frac{(140 - \text{age [years]}) \times \text{weight (kg)} \times F}{\text{SeCr (micromol/litre)}}$$

where F is 1.23 for males and 1.04 for females.

5   A patient has been stabilised on an oral suspension of drug Q at a dose of 200 mg BD.
    In preparation for discharge, the patient needs to be changed onto a tablet formulation of drug Q, what would be the equivalent total daily dose? Give your answer to the nearest whole number.

The bioavailability of drug Q is as follows:

IV = 1
Suspension = 0.6
Tablet = 0.8

6   You have available to you an oral solution containing 4% w/v drug Y and are asked by the nurse to calculate the dose a child needs. The child has been prescribed an oral dose of 50 mg of drug Y TDS.
    What volume of the oral solution do you require for a 5-day course? Give your answer to the nearest whole mL.

7   A patient has visited the warfarin clinic and after checking his INR it is decided to prescribe warfarin 6 mg tonight, followed by alternating daily doses of 3 mg and then 2 mg.
    How many 1 mg warfarin tablets will the pharmacist need to dispense for a 21-day supply?

8   Mr P presents a prescription for prednisolone tablets 5 mg. The initial dose of 40 mg daily is to be taken for 2 weeks. After 2 weeks, he is to reduce his daily dose by 5 mg each week until the course is finished.
    How many 5 mg prednisolone tablets are needed to cover the whole course? Give your answer to the nearest whole number.

9   Ms SB has been diagnosed with rhinitis and prescribed a fluticasone furoate 27.5 micrograms per dose nasal spray. The dose prescribed is TWO sprays to each nostril once daily for two weeks and then reduce to ONE spray in each nostril thereafter.
    If each bottle of fluticasone furoate nasal spray contains 120 doses, how many full bottles of nasal spray do you need to dispense to cover an 8-week supply? Give your answer to the nearest whole number.

10 Mr IS has been prescribed 15 mL carbocisteine 250 mg/5 mL syrup TDS for excessive viscous mucus. He would prefer capsules instead.

Assuming no difference in bioavailability between oral formulations, how many carbocisteine 375 mg capsules would need to be issued to cover a 28-day supply at an equivalent dose to the liquid? Give your answer to the nearest whole number.

11 A syringe driver has been set up to 6 mm/hour to deliver palliative medication to a patient. The length of the syringe driver is 20 cm and it holds 60 mL of injection solution. The injection solution contains 3 micrograms of diamorphine per mL.
How many minutes will it take to deliver 30 micrograms of diamorphine? Give your answer to the nearest ten minutes.

12 What weight, in grams, of calamine powder is required to make 600 g of 4% w/w calamine cream? Give your answer to the nearest whole gram.

13 You are asked to prepare a sterile solution for infusion that contains 350 mg of hydrocortisone which is diluted to 7000 mL with saline for infusion 0.9%.
What is the final concentration of hydrocortisone given as a percentage w/v? Give your answer to three decimal places.

14 You are asked to prepare 250 mL of a disinfectant solution containing 23% v/v phenol, 18% v/v coal tar solution and 59% v/v liquid paraffin. What volume of phenol, in mL, is required to complete this supply? Give your answer to one decimal place.

15 In a trial, 400 men aged 35–85 were treated with a new antihypertensive drug, LowBeePee. Two years later, the death rate from ischaemic heart disease (IHD) was received and the results are given below.

Drug given	Survived	Died
LowBeePee	230	70
Placebo	80	20

Using the formula:

Number needed to treat (NNT) = 100/ARR (absolute risk reduction)

Where AEE = CER (control event rate %) – EER (experimental event rate)

Calculate the NNT for LowBeePee. Give your answer as a whole number.

16 You are a locum working in community pharmacy. The pharmacy chain uses a formula to calculate the price for private prescriptions:

Private prescription cost = (cost of medicine + 20%) + £4.50 dispensing fee per item + £3.50 additional fee for a CD item
Use this formula to calculate the total cost of the following prescription. Give your answer to the nearest whole pound sterling (£).

Drug	Quantity	Cost price
Docusate capsules	100 capsules	£6.84/100 capsules
Tramadol M/R 50 mg capsules	60 capsules	£16.83/60 capsules
Nitromin (glyceryl trinitrate) spray 180 dose	1 bottle	£4.69 per 180 dose bottle

17 You are asked to prepare a dozen paracetamol suppositories each weighing 2 g but containing 250 milligrams of active ingredient using theobroma oil as a base. The displacement value of paracetamol is 1.5. Calculate the quantity of theobroma oil you will need to make twelve suppositories. Give your answer in grams to one decimal place.

18 Calculate the quantity of cocoa butter base required to make 6 × 1.5 g suppositories each containing 300 mg of aspirin (displacement volume 1.1). Give your answer in grams to one decimal place.

19 Calculate the quantity of *Witepsol*® base required to make 21 × 2 g suppositories each containing 250 mg of copper sulfate (displacement volume 3). Give your answer in grams to one decimal place.

20 A patient on your ward has been prescribed sodium chloride infusion 0.9% w/v for electrolyte replacement. The junior doctor on the ward asks you how many mmols of sodium chloride are contained in a 2500 mL bag of the 0.9% w/v solution.
If the RMM of NaCl is 58.5, what is the concentration of sodium chloride in mmol/L? Give your answer to the nearest whole mmol.

21 You are working in an aseptics department and have been requested to prepare a 2.5 L solution containing 8 mmol/L of magnesium ions.
If the molecular weight of magnesium sulphate is 246.5, calculate the volume, in millilitres, of magnesium sulphate 40% w/v needed to produce this solution. Give your answer to one decimal place.

22 You are required to make an IV infusion according to the following formula:

Drug	Concentration (mmol/L)	Molecular weight
Potassium chloride	60	74.5
Sodium bicarbonate	175	84
Sodium chloride	30	58.5

How many grams of sodium bicarbonate are needed to make a 1500 mL infusion? Give your answer to two decimal places.

23 Miss SA is a 34-year-old woman who has been prescribed phenytoin to manage her epilepsy. She has been admitted to hospital and is undergoing investigations for phenytoin toxicity. She currently has an albumin level of 23 g/L and a trough phenytoin concentration of 21 mg/L.
Using the following formula, calculate Miss SA's adjusted phenytoin levels in mg/L. Give your answer to one decimal place.

$$\text{Adjusted phenytoin (mg/L)} = \frac{\text{Measured phenytoin concentration (mg/L)}}{(0.9 \times \text{albumin (g/L)}/42) + 0.1}$$

24 Mr PT, a 47-year-old man, is being treated for hospital-acquired pneumonia with an intravenous infusion of co-amoxiclav. Mr PT has been prescribed a dose of 1.2 g of co-amoxiclav TDS. Each 10 mL vial is diluted with 100 mL saline 0.9% to be infused over 30–60 minutes. What is the maximum rate at which each dose can be administered? Give your answer to two decimal places in mL/minute.

25 You are working on a palliative care ward and are managing a patient who has been prescribed cyclizine 150 mg over 24 hours via a syringe driver to treat severe nausea and vomiting. The cyclizine is available as 50 mg/mL ampoules and the total dose is then diluted to a final volume of 20 mL. The syringe driver available has a length of 5 cm.
Calculate the rate, in mm/hour, the syringe driver needs to be set at to deliver the correct dose to the patient. Give your answer to two decimal places.

26 Mr VD, who weighs 71 kg, has been prescribed an intravenous infusion of dopamine hydrochloride. The dose of dopamine prescribed is at a rate of 2.75 micrograms/kg/min. The hospital pharmacy only has infusion bags of dopamine containing 125 mg per 100 mL.
At what rate, in mL/hr, should the infusion pump be set? Give your answer to one decimal place.

27 Mrs MB has been admitted to the critical care unit and is being kept in a medical coma. Therefore, the patient is unable to swallow any medication. The consultant asks you to calculate an equivalent dose of hydrocortisone 40 mg daily with an injectable formulation of the drug to treat adrenocortical sufficiently in Addison's disease. Hydrocortisone is available as a 5% solution for injection. The bioavailability of tablets is 0.9 and the bioavailability of injection is 1.

How many mLs of this solution for injection should be recommended per day to give a dose equivalent to the oral dose previously taken? Give your answer to two decimal places.

28 You are the lead pharmacist in the specials manufacturing department of a hospital and receive a request for some 4.5% w/v calamine ointment, but the pharmacy only has 1.5% w/v calamine ointment in stock.

Calculate the amount of calamine powder BP in grams that must be added to 450 g of 1.5% w/w calamine ointment to produce a final concentration of 4.5% w/w calamine ointment. Give your answer to two decimal places.

29 A 42-year-old patient weighing 73 kg was prescribed an aminophylline infusion to treat severe acute asthma. He is given aminophylline at a dose of 500 mcg/kg/hour. You are given an infusion bag that contains 25 mg/100 mL.

If one drop is 0.05 mL, calculate the drop rate in drops/minute the infusion is to be set at. Give your answer to the nearest drop/minute.

30 You are presented with the following hospital prescription, written for a 4-year-old child weighing 15 kg:

Date	Infusion	Infusion rate	Prescriber's signature
Today's date	Immunoglobulin 10% 0.3 g/kg	0.75 mL/kg/hr for 45 minutes then: 1.2 mL/kg/hr for 30 minutes then: 1.75 mL/kg/hr for the remainder of the infusion	Dr Ranja Today's date

What is the total infusion duration of the immunoglobulin if infused at the prescribed rate? Give your answer to the nearest whole minute.

31 A 6-year-old child weighing 22 kg is prescribed trimethoprim for prophylaxis of recurrent urinary tract infection. The consultant asks for the trimethoprim to be prescribed at a once daily dose of 2 mg/kg taken at night. You provide the patient's guardian with a 5 mL oral

syringe that is marked in 0.1 mL increments to ensure accurate dosing of this medication.

Calculate the amount of trimethoprim 50 mg/5 mL oral suspension in millilitres the child needs to cover a 28-day course of treatment. Give your answer to the nearest 5 mL.

32 Mr SM has been prescribed idarubicin hydrochloride to treat acute non-lymphocytic leukaemia. The dose is 30 mg/m^2 daily for 3 days.

If Mr SM has a body surface area of 1.33 m^2, calculate how many idarubicin hydrochloride 5 mg capsules are needed to complete this cycle of chemotherapy. Give your answer to the nearest whole capsule.

33 You are working as a pharmacist on the intensive care ward at a local hospital when a doctor has a query regarding a 500 mL infusion of morphine sulphate.

If the infusion contains 40 millimoles of morphine, how many grams of morphine are contained in this infusion? Give your answer in grams to two decimal places.

RMM morphine = 285.3 g/mole.

34 A GP contacts you regarding a patient and their medication, *Accrete*® (calcium carbonate 1500 mg/colecalciferol 10 mcg), taken to prevent osteoporosis. The current dose is *Accrete*® D3 tablets 1 TDS. Each tablet contains 1.5 g calcium carbonate; this is the equivalent of 600 mg of calcium.

The doctor asks you to calculate how many *Calceos*® tablets give an equivalent daily dose. Each *Calceos*® tablet contains 1.25 g calcium carbonate which is equivalent to 500 mg of calcium. Give your answer to the nearest whole tablet.

35 You are working as a GP practice pharmacist and receive a letter from antenatal care from the local hospital. They have recently reviewed a patient, Mrs PR, a 39 year-old who has just been for her first clinic visit. As Mrs PR has a BMI greater than 30, the letter advises that she should take 5 mg folic acid supplement daily during the first trimester of pregnancy. Mrs PR is unable to swallow tablets.

Calculate how much folic acid solution 500 mcg/1 mL needs to be prescribed to cover a 14-day supply. Give your answer to the nearest 10 mL.

36 Ms HP, a female patient aged 55 and weighing 58 kg, has been suffering from meningitis. She is to be treated with benzylpenicillin infusion at a dose of 0.1 g/kg/hour over a 24-hour period. The infusion contains 150,000 mg of benzylpenicillin in 750 mL of normal saline.

What rate should the infusion pump be set at in mL/hour? Give your answer to the nearest whole number.

37 As a specials manufacturing pharmacist you are asked to supply 3500 mL of a concentrated potassium permanganate solution, so that 40 mLs of this diluted to 500 mL would produce a 0.5% w/v solution. What is the weight of potassium permanganate in grams required for the concentrated solution? Give your answer to two decimal places.

38 A 10-year-old child weighing 32 kg has been prescribed flucloxacillin 250 mg/5 mL oral suspension to treat a minor skin abscess. The doctor prescribes a dose of 35 mg/kg each day.
How many days will a 100 mL bottle of flucloxacillin 250 mg/5 mL oral suspension last? Give your answer to the nearest whole day.

39 Mr LS is a 12-year-old who has been diagnosed with severe juvenile active rheumatoid arthritis. The consultant has prescribed methotrexate 15 mg/m^2 to be administered once weekly.
Using the table below, calculate the weekly oral dose in mg suitable for Mr LS. Give your answer to two decimal places.

Age (years)	Body surface area (m^2)
3	0.62
5	0.73
7	0.88
12	1.25

40 Ms SJ is a patient in your hospital ward. She was admitted to treat meningitis and has been prescribed meropenem 2 g every 8 hours. Her serum creatinine is 150 micromol/L. Ms SJ is 82 years old and weighs 49 kg. Creatinine clearance is calculated using the following formula:

$$\text{Creatinine clearance (mL/min)} = \frac{1.04\,(140-\text{age}) \times \text{weight (kg)}}{\text{serum creatinine (micromol/L)}}$$

The SPC recommends the following guidance for the use of meropenem in renal impairment:

Use normal dose every 12 hours	eGFR = 26–50 mL/min/1.73 m^2
Use half normal dose every 12 hours	eGFR = 10–25 mL/min/1.73 m^2
Use half normal dose every 24 hours	eGFR = 10 mL/min/1.73 m^2

Calculate the maximum daily dose in grams SJ can receive considering her level of renal impairment.

SECTION D

Pratik Thakkar

1   You are working for a pharmaceutical company and have a product that is available in tablets and oral suspension. These two products are not dose equivalent as their individual bioavailability is different. A pharmacist rings medical information to ask what the equivalent dose is for a patient taking one 500 mg tablet. The internal data sheet shows the following information on bioavailability:

Tablet bioavailability: 75%
Oral suspension bioavailability: 85%

What is the equivalent dose of the oral suspension (50 mg/mL) needed to maintain at least the same bioavailability? Give your answer to the nearest whole mL.

2   A patient has been admitted to a medical ward for further investigations. The doctor wants to prescribe maintenance fluids. You advise the team to refer to the NICE guidance on intravenous fluid therapy in over 16s in hospital (CG174) and find the following:

Algorithm 3: Routine maintenance

Give maintenance IV fluids
Normal daily fluid and electrolyte requirements

- 1–30 L/kg/day water
- 1 mmol/kg/day sodium and potassium
- 50–100 g/day glucose

The patient has a weight of 65 kg. Your ward stocks glucose 5% bags in volumes of 250 mL, 500 mL, and 1000 mL.
What is the maximum volume of fluid that should be prescribed for that day? Give your answer to the nearest 100 mL.

3   An oncology patient is due to commence a course of methotrexate and his oncologist would like to dose him at 50 mg/m^2. You look at the patient's notes and find that he is 1.70 m tall and weighs 80 kg. Mosterller formula for body surface area:

BSA (m^2) = $\sqrt{([\text{height (cm)} \times \text{weight (kg)}] \div 3600)}$

Calculate the dose of methotrexate that should be prescribed. Give your answer to the nearest milligram.

4   A patient has been admitted to the ward with cardiac failure. She weighs 70 kg and has normal renal function. She is currently taking pravastatin, amlodipine and omeprazole. This is the first time she has been prescribed a cardiac glycoside. The doctor decides to prescribe a total loading dose of 600 mcg.

What is the total volume of digoxin solution needed to be diluted with a diluent for the first portion of the loading dose? Give your answer to one decimal place.

You may use the SPC for Digoxin 250 micrograms/mL Solution for Injection to help you: http://www.medicines.org.uk/emc/medicine/28663

5   You are carrying out a medicines use review for a patient taking warfarin and ask them about what dose they take on a daily basis. They state that they are on two brown tablets and one pink tablet a day. Looking at the BNF, you see the following information:

- 0.5 mg (500 micrograms) – white
- 1 mg – brown
- 3 mg – blue
- 5 mg – pink

What is the daily dose of warfarin the patient is taking? Give your answer to the nearest whole number.

6   Ms R has been diagnosed with pneumonia and needs to be prescribed broad spectrum antibiotics. Before deciding on the dose of an antibiotic, her kidney function needs to be determined. She suffers from chronic kidney disease and her serum creatinine is currently 160 micromol/L. She is 70 years old and weighs 50 kg.

Use the Cockcroft and Gault formula to calculate Ms R's creatinine clearance. Give your answer to two decimal places.

$$\text{CrCl (mL/min)} = \frac{(140 - \text{age [years]}) \times \text{weight (kg)} \times F}{\text{SeCr (micromol/litre)}}$$

where F is 1.23 for males and 1.04 for females.

7   Miss F presents to your pharmacy informing you that she needs magnesium supplements as prescribed by her doctor after she was diagnosed with hypomagnesaemia. The prescription is for magnesium glycerophosphate, two tablets to be taken three times a day as directed. Given that each tablet of magnesium glycerophosphate contains 4 mmol of Mg^{2+}, how much magnesium is Miss F receiving per day? Give your answer to the nearest whole number.

8 A patient has been prescribed aripiprazole 1 mg/mL once a day at a dose of 15 mg/day. The bottle comes in a size of 480 mL.
How many days will one bottle last for? Give your answer to the nearest whole number.

9 You have received an order for 60 g of hydrocortisone/crotamiton cream 2%. Your pharmacy only has the 1% and 2.5% formulations available.
How much of the 1% cream do you need to use in order to make the required cream? Give your answer to the nearest gram.

10 A patient weighing 55 kg presents to the A&E unit with suspected paracetamol poisoning. The clinicians decide to start the patient on acetylcysteine for paracetamol poisoning. Acetylcysteine is available in 10 mL ampoules at a strength of 200 mg/mL.
They follow the Royal College of Emergency Medicine document on the three separate infusions required:

Infusion 1: 150 mg/kg for one hour
Infusion 2: 50 mg/kg over 4 hours
Infusion 3: 100 mg/kg over 16 hours

What are the total number of ampoules to be supplied to treat this case? Give your answer to the nearest whole number.

11 You are extemporaneously preparing morphine sulphate 20 mg suppositories with a base of paraffin. You need to create a batch of 15 morphine sulphate 20 mg suppositories, each weighing 2 g. The displacement value is stated as 1.5.
How much total paraffin is needed as a base for this preparation? Give your answer to three decimal places.

12 A paediatric patient is suffering from hypocalcaemia in the ward. As the parenteral nutrition pharmacist, you decide that the patient would benefit from a separate infusion of calcium 15 mmol over 12 hours. You need to support the nurses to make up an appropriate IV infusion. You find the following molecular masses for compounds commonly used to make up intravenous infusions including parenteral nutrition.

Formula	g/mol
$CaCl_2 \cdot 2H_2O$	147.01
KCl	74.55
$MgCl_2$	95.21
NaCl	58.44

How many millilitres of calcium chloride injection BP (calcium chloride dihydrate) solution 14.7% w/v should be used in this infusion? Give your answer to the nearest millilitre.

13 You are at a palliative care home and are reviewing a patient's drug chart and note that he is currently taking two *MST Continus*® 30 mg sachets twice a day. However, after speaking to the patient, he is starting to experience regular breakthrough pain and you need to advise on an appropriate dose of *Oramorph*® 10 mg/5 mL to manage his pain. What is the minimum dose of PRN *Oramorph*® solution, as per BNF guidelines, that can be prescribed for an episode of breakthrough pain for this patient? Give your answer to the nearest whole number.

14 You are helping a respiratory physician create a dosing schedule for prednisolone with a weaning dose for COPD exacerbations. Based on historical practice, patients start their reducing schedule as follows: 30 mg once a day for 5 days, then wean by 5 mg every 3 days until finished. How many 5 mg prednisolone tablets should be supplied to ensure patients can complete this weaning course? Give your answer to the nearest whole tablet.

15 You are extemporaneously preparing aqueous calamine cream and have the instruction sheet as follows:

The ingredients include:

- calamine 4% w/w
- zinc oxide 3% w/w
- glyceryl monostearate 1% w/w
- macrogol cetostearyl 2% w/w
- liquid paraffin made up to 100 g

How much liquid paraffin will you need to make 250 g of the cream? Give your answer to the nearest whole number.

16 You are a paediatric pharmacist and are reviewing a patient's fluid balance. The patient is to be put on full maintenance fluid regimen per day as per the doctor's advice. The patient weighs 36 kg. The maintenance fluid can be calculated using the following formula as per the BNFC:

- 100 mL/kg for first 10 kg body weight, plus
- 50 mL/kg for next 10 kg, plus
- 20 mL/kg for each kg thereafter up to max of 70 kg

How much fluid can this patient have in 24 hours? Give your answer to the nearest whole millilitre.

17   A 2-month-old baby attends the GP practice for their routine child-
     hood immunisations. The GP would like to prescribe paracetamol
     suppositories for the child in case they develop a fever.
     What is the maximum number of suppositories the child can use in a
     24-hour period? Give your answer to the nearest whole number.
     You may use the SPC for *Alvedon*® Suppositories 60 mg to help you:
     https://www.medicines.org.uk/emc/product/3698/smpc

18   You are on the intensive care unit reviewing patients' notes. A patient's
     drug chart is missing from the bed and you urgently need to work out
     the dose of dobutamine a patient is receiving. The reading on a syringe
     driver administering dobutamine is 42 mL/hr. The infusion volume
     is 500 mL at a concentration of 0.05% w/v of dobutamine solution.
     The patient weighs 60 kg.
     What dose of dobutamine is the patient receiving in microgram/kg/min?
     Give your answer to one decimal place.

19   You are working for a pharmaceutical specials company and are
     required to send 200 mL of an antiseptic solution which when diluted
     1 in 20 produces a 1 mg in 5 mL solution. The concentrate of the
     antiseptic is available at a strength of 50% w/v.
     What volume of the concentrate is needed to fulfil this order? Give your
     answer to one decimal place.

20   An injection solution of tirofiban contains 250 mcg/ml of active ingredi-
     ent. A hospital manufacturing unit is creating batches of 1 mL injection
     solution in ampoules for supply to its wards and to other hospitals.
     Each batch size is 400 ampoules plus 1% extra ampoules for QC batch
     testing.
     How much tirofiban powder is needed to prepare two batches worth?
     Give your answer to the nearest whole number.

21   A 75-year-old male patient recently received a loading dose of 500 mcg
     and the doctor has decided to maintain him on digoxin IV. The patient's
     serum creatinine level is 95 μmol/L. You work out the maintenance
     dose for digoxin.
     What is the maintenance dose of digoxin, in mcg, as calculated? Give
     your answer to the nearest whole number.
     You may use the SPC for Digoxin 250 micrograms/ml Solution for Injec-
     tion to help you: https://www.medicines.org.uk/emc/product/5290/smpc

22   You have been asked to calculate the rate for an infusion of 150 mg
     morphine in 1 L of glucose 5% at a rate of 60 mcg/kg/hr for a 57 kg
     female patient.

Assuming 20 drops per mL, what is the nearest approximate whole drop rate per minute that needs to be set on the giving set? Give your answer to the nearest whole number.

23 A patient requires some phenobarbitone for seizure control. The instructions require the product to be added to glucose 5%. When vials of phenobarbitone powder for solution for infusion are reconstituted, the resultant solution is 1% in 40 mL.
Assuming no displacement, to what volume of glucose 5% must the 40 mL solution of phenobarbitone 1% w/v be added, in order to produce a 0.2% w/v solution? Give your answer to the nearest millilitre.

24 A 6-year-old patient weighing 18 kg presents to A&E with a high grade fever and non-blanching rash. The doctors suspect that the patient has acute bacterial meningitis. They follow local microbiology guidelines and are required to administer meropenem. The nurses would like to reconstitute the product to 50 mL of 0.9% sodium chloride.
What is the concentration of the final dose to be given for infusion? Give your answer to two decimal places.
You may use the SPC for meropenem IV to help you: https://www.medicines.org.uk/emc/product/6731/smpc

25 You are working with your health economics and outcomes research colleague to work out the impact a new product may have for breast cancer. For a genetically defined mutation sub-population of breast cancer patients, you have been told that the average utility value for these patients is 0.5, and they usually survive for 14 months if they receive best supportive care. The new product, through clinical trials in breast cancer in patients who had the same genetically defined mutation, has shown an increased utility value of 0.7 and the patients survived for an average of 37 months.
What is the difference in quality adjusted life years (QALY) with the new product versus the best supportive care available? Give your answer to one decimal place.

QALY = years of life × utility value

26 A patient presents to the pharmacy and would like to buy *Acidex Advance*® Oral Suspension (aniseed flavour). They need to take this medication for acid reflux. You note that they should be on a sodium-controlled diet which they are recommended to be on a maximum of 2 g of sodium a day. The atomic mass of sodium is 23. The product contains 5 mmol of sodium per 10 mL dose.

What percentage of daily sodium allowance is the patient receiving from the product if they take two doses a day? Give your answer to one decimal place.

27 You work for the PK analysis team in a pharmaceutical company and need to work out the dose for a patient in a trial using the pharmacokinetic profile of one of the products in development.
The patient weighs 70 kg and has no past medical history. Below is a basic product pharmacokinetic profile for information:

Product × profile
Oral tablet
Pharmacokinetic model: Single compartment open model
Bioavailability: 70%
Volume of distribution (Vd) = 0.4 L/kg
Dose = Vd × plasma level

A plasma level that is desired for the team is to reach 6.2 mg/L. Assuming the patient needs to only take one dose, what is the oral dose required to reach this level? Give your answer to the nearest 10 mg.

28 A patient is being discharged from the ward and has, amongst other conditions, otitis externa infection. The clinician has prescribed the patient to take gentamicin with hydrocortisone drops as per local guidelines. The recommended dose is: 2–4 drops QDS for 7 days. The gentamicin HC bottles come in 10 mL volumes.
Assuming 20 drops per mL, how many bottles should be supplied if the patient is to use the maximum dose permitted? Give your answer to the nearest whole bottle.

29 You are calculating the cost difference between different treatment regimens for *Helicobacter pylori* eradication. Your practice currently prefers to use the following regimen: omeprazole 20 mg BD, clarithromycin 250 mg BD and metronidazole 400 mg BD (7-day course). You would like to review the following regimen to determine if it would be cheaper: esomeprazole 20 mg OD, amoxicillin 1 g BD and clarithromycin 500 mg BD (7-day course).
The following are the costs of the products:

Product	Cost
Esomeprazole 20 mg tablets (28 tablets)	£2.24
Omeprazole 20 mg capsules (28 capsules)	£5.55
Amoxicillin 500 mg capsules (21 capsules)	£1.15
Clarithromycin 250 mg tablets (14 tablets)	£1.30
Metronidazole tablets (21 tablets)	£4.10

How much cheaper is a 7-day course of esomeprazole, amoxicillin and clarithromycin compared to the existing regimen used in your pharmacy? Give your answer to the nearest 10 pence.

30 A patient is on a course of gemcitabine monotherapy for non-small cell lung cancer. For his first cycle, the regimen was followed as normal. After the weeks rest, he presented with granulocytosis and the results of the blood test show that he has a granulocyte count of 990×10^6/L and a platelet count of $65,000 \times 10^6$/L. The patient's basic characteristics are as follows: height = 1.6 m, weight = 72 kg.

BSA (m^2) = $\sqrt{}$ ([height (cm) × weight (kg)] ÷ 3600)

What is the next calculated dose for the patient considering the resource below and the information above? Give your answer to the nearest 10 mg.
You may use the SPC for Gemcitabine 1 g powder for solution for infusion to help you: https://www.medicines.org.uk/emc/product/2490/smpc

31 You visit an American industrial manufacturing site that produces active pharmaceutical ingredients for the products that your company manufactures. One of the drums contains 250 L of concentrated product Y at 22,000 ppm. You need to find out how much product you need to purchase to make a batch of this product at your facility. Each batch of this product at your facility is made of 110 × 250 mL bottles, each containing 25% w/v.
How much concentrated solution of product Y do you need to produce one batch of product Y at your facility plus 10% overage? Give your answer to two decimal places.

32 You are asked to provide potassium permanganate 400 mg tablets for a patient for wound washing.
What is the resultant concentration of the final solution if the patient dissolves two tablets into 250 mL of water, which is then diluted 1 in 40 to produce a bath for washing multiple wounds? Give your answer to three decimal places.

33 You have a palliative care paediatric patient who is on morphine sulphate modified-release tablets at a dose of 30 mg BD. The patient weighs 43 kg and does not take any breakthrough pain medication. The patient cannot take oral medications anymore so you are asked to work out the dosing rate for the clinician to assess whether it is an appropriate dose via an IV route. The BNF states that the parenteral morphine is half the dose of oral morphine.

What is the equivalent dose in mcg/kg/hour for parenteral infusion? Give your answer to the nearest mcg.

34 You are working with a commissioning GP consortium and are reviewing the use of antipsychotics in your region. The use of *Biquelle XL®* (quetiapine fumarate) has increased recently. Currently, there are 500 patients using this product for schizophrenia. Below is a table of the breakdown of doses of the patients on *Biquelle XL®* for schizophrenia:

Dose of quetiapine slow release per day	Number of patients
800 mg	120
600 mg	250
400 mg	130

There is a newly accepted cheaper alternative available on the regions formulary: *Mintreleq XL®* (quetiapine fumarate). Below are the prices of the tablets:

Strength	Biquelle XL®	Mintreleq XL®
300 mg tablet (60 tablets)	£74.45	£49.99
400 mg tablet (60 tablets)	£98.95	£64.99

What are the potential daily savings the region can make if all patients changed to *Mintreleq XL®*? Give your answer to the nearest 10 pounds.

35 Focusing on the 120 patients on 800 mg *Biquelle XL®*, you discuss this with the clinicians and they advise that there is potential for a few patients on 800 mg dose to be reduced down to the recommended dose if clinically suitable after a consultation with their GP. The BNF states that the recommended daily dose for this product is 600 mg per day. You are tasked to calculate the potential daily savings of *Biquelle XL®* usage if 40% of the high dose patients were reduced to the maintenance dose of 600 mg *Biquelle XL®*. Give your answer to the nearest 10 pounds.

Single best answers

SECTION A

1 B

All beta-blockers are contraindicated in severe peripheral arterial disease. However, abrupt withdrawal of any beta-blockers could exacerbate ischaemic heart disease. Slow the reduction in dose and then stop should be advised.

2 E

ACE inhibitors or a low-cost angiotensin-II receptor blocker are the most appropriate for a person less than 55 years old. Refer to NICE hypertensive guidance.

3 D

See BNFC monograph for paracetamol.

4 D

A long-acting peakless insulin is appropriate in people with hyperglycaemia through the day and night.

5 E

Hypoglycaemia blood glucose concentration is less than 4 mmol/L and in patients with diabetes can cause unresponsiveness.

6 C

See BNF introductory information to chapter 6, section 3.1 for information on diabetes – type 1 diabetes. Hypoglycaemia in diabetes mellitus can be caused by the administration of insulin or sulphonylurea. This can be compounded by impairment of the counter-regulatory response to hypoglycaemia due to secretion of glucagon and adrenaline. Metformin does not cause hypoglycaemia alone; in this case it is due to gliclazide. See SPC for gliclazide 80 mg tablets.

7 B

See BNF introductory information to chapter 6, section 3.2 for information on hypoglycaemia. If no IV access intramuscular glucagon can be administered. This works by stimulating gluconeogenesis and glycogenolysis and is faster acting, easier and quicker to administer than IV glucose.

8 B

Dipeptidyl peptidase-4 inhibitors (DDP-4) cause little or no weight gain, exhibit relatively little risk of hypoglycaemia and have relatively modest glucose-lowering activity.

9 C

Naproxen is the most likely to have caused GI irritation as it was only started 2 weeks ago.
Atorvastatin can cause GI side effects but the patient has taken this for 3 years and so this is unlikely to be the cause of the symptoms.

10 E

Refer to RCOG guidelines for thrombosis and embolism during pregnancy and the puerperium: acute management: https://www.rcog .org.uk/en/guidelines-research-services/guidelines/gtg37b/. Thrombosis and embolism during LMWH is eliminated more rapidly in pregnancy than in non-pregnant state. LMWH should be administered 12-hourly, rather than daily and monitored to guide dosage adjustment

11 E

See BNF, chapter 2, section 3.2 – introduction on heparins. Clinically important heparin-induced thrombocytopenia is immune-mediated and can be complicated by thrombosis. Signs of heparin-induced thrombocytopenia include a 30% reduction of platelet count, thrombosis, or skin allergy.

12 C

See BNF monograph for phenytoin.

13 B

See BNF monograph for phenytoin. The current dosage seems to yield a serum phenytoin concentration that is lower than what we are seeking to achieve (the upper half of the target range i.e. 15–20 microgram/mL) so the dosage should be increased. Phenytoin is a drug with a narrow therapeutic index i.e. little margin of safety between dose required for therapeutic effect and the dose that may be toxic, thus monitoring of drug concentration is required. Phenytoin possesses zero order kinetics - this means the half will lengthen in proportion to the serum concentration, so dose changes should occur in small increments.

14 C

Phenytoin sodium molecular equivalents are not necessarily biologically equivalent. 100 mg of phenytoin sodium is approximately equivalent in therapeutic effect to 92 mg phenytoin base.

15 E

See BNF, chapter 2, section 4.1 – drugs affecting the renin-angiotensin system. Patient presented with a fall and had symptoms and signs of hypotension. You should withhold ramipril as she continues to have features of hypotension. It may be appropriate to reintroduce later at a lower dose and close monitoring.

16 A

Naproxen would increase the risk of GI bleeding.

17 D

The priority would be to stop her naproxen because it could worsen her existing renal impairment and increase gastrointestinal and cardiovascular risk further.

18 C

Colchicine is an alternative in patients in whom NSAIDs are contraindicated. Aspirin is not indicated in gout. Allopurinol is not effective in treating an acute attack and can prolong it indefinitely if started during the acute episode. Patient has heart failure thus value in patients with heart failure since, unlike NSAIDs, it does not induce fluid retention.

ANSWERS

19 B

Thiazide diuretics can raise the serum urate level. It is probably better to avoid thiazides in patients with coexistent gout and hypertension.

20 D

Maintain the same dose and increase the dosage interval. The half-life of gentamicin is short, approximately 2.5 hours, thus 2.5 hours after dose is administered only 50% of the dose should remain. After 20 hours after the dose, almost none should remain, thus trough should be very low (<1 mg/L). If not, drug is being eliminated more slowly than anticipated. To reduce further nephrotoxicity, it would be preferable to withhold the second dose until the previous one has been eliminated.

21 E

Refer to NICE guidance on chronic obstructive pulmonary disease in over 16s: diagnosis and management (NG115).

22 B

See BNFC, Medical emergencies in the community, Anaphylaxis. Adrenaline is an important drug that is used in a number of emergency medical situations. It is the first-line treatment for severe allergic reactions (anaphylaxis).

23 E

The bacteria most likely to cause COPD exacerbations are *haemophilus influenza, moraxella catarrhalis, streptococcus pneumoniae*. Refer to NICE COPD guide or Global Initiative for Chronic Obstructive Lung Disease.

24 D

Relvar Ellipta® is a combination medicinal product (long-acting beta$_2$-agonist (vilanterol) and inhaled corticosteroid (fluticasone furoate). During inhalation corticosteroids can deposit inside the mouth and cause fungal infection. It is advised to rinse the mouth after using inhalers that contain steroids.

25 A

First-line antibiotics in COPD exacerbation include tetracyclines, amoxicillin and macrolides. These are broad-spectrum antibiotics.

26 D

Olanzapine is a dopamine D_1, D_2, D_4, 5-HT_2 histamine- 1-, and muscarinic-receptor antagonist. An ECG may be required, particularly if physical examination identifies cardiovascular risk factors, personal history of cardiovascular disease, or if the patient is being admitted as an inpatient. See: https://www.formularycomplete.com/view/drug/monograph/49776

27 C

See BNF, chapter 2, section 4.1 – hypertension in pregnancy. Only licensed products should be used in pregnancy for hypertension. First-line is labetalol if not contraindicated (oral or intravenous).

28 E

Refer to WHO pain ladder. Patient is on treatment step for moderate-to-severe pain, but need to optimise by adding in a sustained release morphine sulphate (*MST Continus*®).

29 D

This patient was prescribed *Oramorph*® morphine sulphate 10 mg in 5 ml; 2.5 mg every 2 hours, thus 12×2.5 mg dose of the short-acting morphine in 24 hours (a total of 30 mg in 24 hours). However, the short-acting morphine is not controlling her pain and doesn't last long. Therefore, prescribing a sustained-release preparation which is equivalent to the total daily dose of the immediate-release in two divided doses will ensure good background pain relief.

30 B

Dose: $10 \times 2 = 20$ micrograms/min; as the rate is in hours (0.2 mL/hr), convert the dose to hours.
$20 \times 60 = 1200$ micrograms/hr
Syringe is 50 mL, so $50/0.2 = 250$
Multiply by dose to find out how many micrograms in 50 mL
$250 \times 1200 = 300\,000$ mcg = 300 mg
Dobutamine is available as 12.5 mg/mL: $300/12.5 = 24$ mL

31 B

Sodium chloride 0.9% = 0.9 g in 100 mL
$0.9 \times 5 = 4.5$ g in 500 mL
Sodium chloride 30% = 30 g in 100 mL
4.5 g is needed: $(4.5/30) \times 100 = 15$ mL

32 A

The rash is contagious, itchy and mainly presents on the face and spread across the back in clusters of small red lumps and some fluid-filled vesicles.

33 C

See Community Pharmacy: Symptoms, Diagnosis and Treament, 2nd ed., Rutter. Chickenpox is a viral infection caused by the varicella-zoster virus (VZV).

34 C

This child weighs 12 kg.
100 mL/kg/day × 10 kg = 1000 mL/ day
50 mL/kg/day × 2 kg = 100 mL/day
20 mL/kg/day x 0 kg = 0 mL/day
Thus maintenance fluid = 1100 mL/day

35 E

5 × 12 × 10 = 600 mL

36 E

Daily fluid requirement = maintenance + deficit
1100 mL + 600 mL = 1700 mL

37 A

See BNF, chapter 14, section 4.

38 A

Although the patient is less than 55 years of age, his age, ethnicity and comorbidities need to be considered. NICE advises in a black person of African or Caribbean origin first-line treatment is to initiate a calcium channel blocker. Refer to NICE hypertension guidance: https://pathways.nice.org.uk/pathways/hypertension/hypertension-overview#content=view-index&path=view%3a/pathways/hypertension/treatment-steps-for-hypertension.xml

39 C

See BNF, chapter 2, section 4.1 – calcium-channel blockers. Calcium-channel blockers like amlodipine cause side-effects associated with vasodilatation, such as flushing and headache (which becomes less obtrusive after a few days), and ankle swelling – these are all common side-effects.

40 E

See BNF, Appendix 1 Interactions – trimethoprim and BNF monograph for methotrexate. Prescribing error occurred because it is not appropriate to prescribe trimethoprim to a person receiving methotrexate because of a serious and potentially life-threatening increased risk of haematological toxicity. Serious drug interaction causes bone marrow suppression and nephrotoxicity. Both agents inhibit dihydrofolate reductase, the combination of these two drugs substantially reduces folate metabolism and increases the potential for myelosuppression. Both sulphonamides and methotrexate have the potential to cause nephrotoxicity, and the resulting renal impairment can itself lead to increased levels of either or both drugs.

SECTION B

1 C

PPIs are implicated in increasing risk of *C. difficile* infection and should be withheld during episodes of *C. difficile* infection.

2 C

Numerous anticonvulsants and antidepressants can cause hyponatraemia, which can manifest as confusion.

3 B

SGLT2 inhibitors are known to cause euglycemic DKA.

4 B

Intravenous is the only route vincristine should be administered. Vinka alkaloids must not be given intrathecally due to risk of death, or subcutaneously due to tissue necrosis.

5 A

See BNF monograph for folic acid. Folic acid should not be taken on the same day as methotrexate. It is generally taken on any other day.

6 B

See BNF introductory information to chapter 4, section 3.4 for information on antidepressant drugs – monoamine-oxidase inhibitors. At least one week should be left between stopping TCAs and commencing a MAOI.

7 B

All the other foods are associated with higher levels of tyramine, which can lead to hypertensive conditions and crises in patients taking non-reversible MOAIs like phenelzine.

8 E

This is a well-known interaction between phenelzine and venlafaxine. Pharmacists should know what drugs can cause serotonin syndrome and how to identify this. They should also be able to help medical teams distinguish between this and neuroleptic malignant syndrome.

9 E
Patients must be warned of the risks of phototoxicity and how
to avoid this. Tablets can be crushed and dispersed if the patient
struggles to swallow tablets. Microdeposits in the eye are fairly
common but do not always cause glare with headlights and patient
should not be told to avoid driving unless this happens. See SPC,
section 4.4 Special warnings and precautions for use.

10 C
Patients of Afro-Caribbean descent should be offered a calcium
channel blocker alongside an ACE inhibitor. Refer to NICE guidance
on type 2 diabetes mellitus (NIDDM) regarding the management
of hypertension: https://www.nice.org.uk/guidance/ng28/chapter/1-
Recommendations#blood-pressure-management-2

11 C
Patients with an FEV_1 greater than 50% of predicted should be
offered a LAMA or LABA. A LAMA is preferred over a SAMA
at this stage of treatment. Patients using a SAMA for relief should
stop taking this if given a LAMA. Steroids are only licensed in
combination with a LAMA and should only be used if FEV_1 is less
than 50% predicted, or a LAMA or LABA hasn't improved the
condition. Candidates should read the overview in the BNF or refer
to the NICE/GOLD guidance.

12 E
National Guidance (from NHS and St John Ambulance) is to perform
30 chest compressions then give two rescue breaths.

13 A
Broccoli can cause blockages in a stoma as it is high in fibre. This
said, all ileostomates should be advised to eat healthily but have small
mouthfuls and chew their food well. More information is available
on NHS Choices: https://www.nhs.uk/conditions/ileostomy/living-
with/

14 B
Thiazide diuretics are known to cause hyperglycaemia.

ANSWERS

15 A

See BNF advice on vomiting in pregnancy. This patient is in the first trimester, so her nausea should be self-limiting and active treatment is generally not necessary.

16 C

See BNF monograph for carbimazole and notes on neutropenia and agranulocytosis. This patient needs to be referred to her GP for further investigations.

17 C

See MEP 42, Appendix 5 GPhC in practice: guidance on raising concerns. You should report concerns to your line manager, and/or the line manager of the pharmacist you have a concern about, or someone else within the organisation before reporting it to the GPhC.

18 E

See MEP 42, section 3.5 Veterinary medicines. As this product is licenced for use in this disease in this species, it is not necessary to follow the veterinary prescribing cascade.

19 A

See BNFC notes on diarrhoea and oral rehydration therapy. Anti-motility drugs not recommended in children under 12 years of age. The patient in question is not at significant risk of dehydration given age and clinical timeline.

20 B

Introduction to chapter 5 in the BNF states that clarithromycin can be used in those with penicillin allergy. Note the presence of beta-lactam rings in cephalosporin and carbapenem structures.

21 A

See BNF information on statin therapy. Atorvastatin is a longer acting statin so may be taken at any time of day. Compare dosing instructions in monographs for simvastatin and atorvastatin.

22 B

See SPC, section 4.2 Posology and method of administration. Creatine phosphokinase (CPK) must be taken before and during treatment to detect any muscle damage.

23 B

See BNF information for loop diuretics. Furosemide can be given twice a day but its duration of action is 6 hours. Therefore, it should not usually be given any later than 4pm.

24 C

See BNF information regarding thiazide diuretics, which may precipitate gout.

25 C

See BNF monograph for lithium. See serum concentration notes for lithium for list of overdose signs and symptoms. See SPC, section 4.9 Overdose for more information.

26 A

See BNF, Appendix 1 and Stockley's Drug Interactions. Amiodarone inhibits the metabolism of coumarin anticoagulants.

27 E

See BNF monograph for aciclovir. Aciclovir cream should be applied to the skin 5 times per day, approximately every 4 hours.

28 C

See BNF introductory information to chapter 11 regarding the application of eye drops and eye ointments, which states 5 minutes interval is advised.

29 C

IV paracetamol should be dosed at 15 mg/kg when patients weigh less than 50 kg. Therefore 630 mg is the maximum dose advised.

30 E

See BNF monographs for quinolones, including levofloxacin, which describes increased risk of tendon damage in those taking corticosteroids. While the patient in this question is not at increased risk of aortic aneurysm, pharmacists should be aware of this new warning: https://www.gov.uk/drug-safety-update/systemic-and-inhaled-fluoroquinolones-small-increased-risk-of-aortic-aneurysm-and-dissection-advice-for-prescribing-in-high-risk-patients

ANSWERS

31 D
Refer to NICE guidance for treatment of lower UTI, and PHE guidelines for management of UTI in primary care. Patient has recently had trimethoprim so is at increased risk of resistance. First-line treatment is nitrofurantoin.

32 A
P values less than 0.05 generally indicates there is a statistically significant difference between two comparators.

33 C
See BNF, chapter 6, section 3.1 for information on diabetic ketoacidosis management. Normal basal insulin should be continued alongside fluids and fixed rate insulin.

34 D
See SPC, section 4.3 Contraindications. Patients with active infections, especially severe infections such as pneumonia causing sepsis and hospitalisation, should not take methotrexate due to its immunosuppressive effects.

35 B
50:50 contains liquid paraffin and white soft paraffin so poses an ignition risk. Trainees should read the warnings from DH and the BNF. When used as a bath additive the ointment should be added to the bath water. If used as a soap substitute it should not be applied to dry skin.

SECTION C

1 E

Ramipril 10 mg OD initiated at a dose too high can cause hypotension.

2 B

A is inappropriate as no bruising or bleeding; C is omitting warfarin for too long; D is incorrect because reducing green vegetables will increase INR and E is an inappropriate referral.

3 B

Diuretics can precipitate lithium toxicity.

4 B

Citalopram 30 mg can prolong QT interval, the other medications cannot.

5 C

ACE inhibitors are the main cause of AKI.

6 C

See BNF monograph for diltiazem hydrochloride. Brand prescribing not required for all other medication; different versions of S/R preparations containing more than 60 mg of diltiazem hydrochloride may not have the same clinical effect, therefore prescribers should specify the brand to be dispensed.

7 B

See BNF information on beta-adrenoceptor blocking drugs. Beta-blockers can affect carbohydrate metabolism, causing hypoglycaemia or hyperglycaemia in patients with or without diabetes; they can also interfere with metabolic and autonomic responses to hypoglycaemia, thereby masking symptoms such as tachycardia. Note – hypoglycaemia is not associated with metformin or alogliptin.

8 A

See BNF monograph for alogliptin. Stop alogliptin due to risk of pancreatitis.

9 **A**
Refer to GP – do not issue miconazole gel as there is a potentially dangerous interaction if the gel is administered whilst taking warfarin.

10 **D**
Refer to NICE stroke guidance and Royal College of Physicians.

11 **E**
To ensure dose is correct you need the baseline for creatinine, weight, urea and electrolytes and liver function tests – see SPC for *Eliquis*® 2.5 mg film-coated tablets. NICE Clinical Knowledge Summaries, Anticoagulation, Oral also recommend baseline full blood count.

12 **E**
SSRIs can cause hyponatraemia and increase the risk of drowsiness/convulsions/confusion in elderly patients.

13 **A**
See MEP 42, section 3.3.12 Supplying isotretinoin and pregnancy prevention.

14 **B**
See BNF monograph for amiodarone.

15 **E**
See BNF monograph for simvastatin.

16 **C**
Refer to NICE guidance for cardiovascular disease: risk assessment and reduction, including lipid modification: https://www.nice.org.uk/guidance/cg181/chapter/1-Recommendations#lipid-modification-therapy-for-the-primary-and-secondary-prevention-of-cvd-2

17 **E**
A is incorrect as patient is penicillin allergic; B is incorrect as there is caution in children due to tendon damage risk; C is incorrect as it contains a penicillin and D is incorrect because all tetracyclines are contraindicated for patients under the age of 12.

18 A
There is interaction between trimethoprim and methotrexate and interaction between pivmecillinam and methotrexate – can use nitrofurantoin cautiously at this renal function.

19 E
See BNF monograph for paroxetine. Paroxetine is associated with a higher risk of withdrawal symptoms if stopped abruptly.

20 A
Amitriptyline is associated with the highest fatality in overdose. Trazodone is related but has less effects and lofepramine is a TCA with least associated complications in comparison to others.

21 D
Intercourse took place 74 hours ago; levonorgestrel is licensed for use within 72 hours. D is the correct dose for ulipistral which is licensed for use within 120 hours.

22 B
As per NICE guidance, more restricted BP targets.

23 A
Glucocorticoids may increase blood glucose levels.

24 C
See BNF monograph for methotrexate. Recommended monitoring of liver function tests, creatinine and full blood count.

25 C
See BNF monograph for pioglitazone. Refer to MHRA/CHM advice.

26 E
Patients need to be on a pregnancy prevention programme. Refer to MHRA.

27 D
See BNF monograph for amlodipine.

28 B
Pharmacists can make the diagnosis for migraine. See RPS OTC sumatriptan guide.

ANSWERS

29 A

No breaks with this therapy. All the rest are correct statements with regards to HRT. See SPC for *Elleste duet*® 1 mg.

30 D

See MEP 42, section 3.3.10.2 Emergency supply. Emergency supplies at the request of a prescriber do not include schedule 1, 2 or 3 controlled drugs.

31 D

See BNF, Appendix 1 Interactions. To avoid together if possible – sildenafil only contraindicated in recent unstable angina.

32 B

See BNF, Prescribing in palliative care. S/C dose is approximately equivalent to half of oral dose.

33 A

Symptoms indicative of bacterial infection so offer item suitable for this age.

34 A

A calcium channel blocker is suitable for this patient. Refer to NICE hypertension guidance, Treatment steps for hypertension: https://pathways.nice.org.uk/pathways/hypertension#path=view% 3A/pathways/hypertension/treatment-steps-for-hypertension.xml& content=view-index

35 E

See BNF monograph for doxycycline. Cautionary and advisory labels 6, 9, 11 and 27 – all apply. E is cautionary advisory label 14 'This medicine may colour your urine. This is harmless.' which does not apply.

36 D

This only applies to the MUR service (http://psnc.org.uk/services-commissioning/advanced-services/murs/national-target-groups-for-murs/), whereas all other options relate to the NMS service (https:// psnc.org.uk/services-commissioning/advanced-services/nms/nms-medicines-list/).

37 A
See BNF, Appendix 1 Interactions.

38 B
Bisoprolol most commonly associated with cold extremities/paraesthesia.

39 D
There is a side effect of hyperglycaemia with diabetes. Therefore if the patient has diabetes they should be encouraged to monitor blood glucose. Steroids should also be used with caution in patients with diabetes.

40 C
See BNF section for bisphosphonates/MHRA/CHM guidelines.

41 B
See BNF, chapter 7, section 3 for information on progestogen-only contraceptives. Progestogen-only pill is a suitable alternative to combined oral contraceptive pill.

42 B
See BNF monograph for finasteride and MHRA/CDM guidelines.

43 B
See MEP 42, section 3.5 Veterinary medicines. All others are legally required.

44 E
See BNF monograph for clozapine. SPC for *Clozaril*® 25 mg and 100 mg tablets states blood pressure should be monitored during the first weeks of treatment.

45 A
This is used to decide appropriate warfarin therapy or DOAC. B and C are bleed scores; D is for heart failure classification and E is a score for statin therapy.

SECTION D

1 A

Bendroflumethiazide is a thiazide diuretic which can cause hypokalaemia by increasing renal excretion of potassium, whereas an ACEI can cause hyperkalaemia.

2 B

Only a minority of this increase is due to the presence of gene mutations. However, the patient should be referred directly to a specialist genetics service if a high-risk predisposing gene mutation has been identified. Refer to NICE CKS Breast cancer – Managing FH: https://cks.nice.org.uk/breast-cancer-managing-fh#!scenariorecommendation:1/-401112

3 E

Oral steroids such as prednisolone inhibit gastric secretion and predispose to ulceration.

4 E

The patient is showing signs of renal failure which is supported by the high levels of creatinine. Ramipril is an ACE inhibitor and reduces angiotensin-II production necessary for preserving glomerular filtration when renal blood flow is reduced.

5 B

See SPC for finasteride 1 mg tablets. Finasteride 1 mg is indicated for the treatment of the first stage of hair loss (androgenic alopecia) in males. Finasteride 1 mg stabilises the process of androgenic alopecia in 18–41 year old males. It is not indicated for use in women or children.

6 A

For pregnant women with epilepsy 5 mg of folic acid should be prescribed. For non-epileptic women the dose of folic acid for pregnant women is 400 mcg.

7 C

Omitting warfarin should cause a decline in the INR levels to reach target levels. Clarithromycin is a macrolide antibiotic and is an enzyme inhibitor which has increased warfarin plasma levels by inhibiting its breakdown.

8 E
Withdraw anti-epileptics one at a time if on a multiple regime.

9 B
Pityriasis versicolor can sometimes be confused with vitiligo since they both cause the skin to become discoloured in patches. However, vitiligo often develops symmetrically on both sides of your body simultaneously, whereas pityriasis versicolor may not develop in a simultaneous or symmetrical fashion. The skin affected by pityriasis versicolor is usually slightly scaly or flaky, whereas in vitiligo there is usually no change to the texture of the skin. Vitiligo is more common around the mouth, eyes, fingers, wrists, armpits and groin, whereas pityriasis versicolor tends to develop on the chest, tummy, back and upper arms.

10 B
Assessment for signs of suicidal ideation is important, especially in the beginning of treatment. Efficacy, however, cannot be determined as early as two weeks into treatment.

11 C
Fatigue is associated with propranolol.

12 C
Pharmacists are also required to undertake the disability assessment under the Equality Act, and in this case due to the number of medicines the patient is taking, a blister pack may help to reduce confusion. Memory should also be monitored for early signs of dementia.

13 C
Diclofenac is an NSAID and can cause acute kidney injury by reducing renal hydraulic pressure and perfusion. Avoid prescribing ACE inhibitors and NSAIDs together, particularly in elderly patients who already have renal impairment to some degree.

14 E
Trimethoprim and methotrexate are both folate antagonists. It is contraindicated to take these concomitantly as it may lead to additive toxicity manifesting in bone marrow suppression and neutropenic sepsis.

ANSWERS

15 B
It is recommended that patients suffering from hypoglycaemia consume 4–5 dextrose tablets or 15–20 g of glucose and retest blood glucose after 10–15 minutes. If the reading is at 4 mmol or above and the patient feels better they should then eat a meal containing carbohydrates. If it's still below 4 mmol, treat again with a sugary drink or snack and take another reading in 10–15 minutes.

16 C
A full blood count including a neutrophil count is important to determine if the sore throat is caused by carbimazole-inducing bone marrow suppression and thus agranulocytosis.

17 E
Simvastatin is contraindicated during pregnancy. Treatment should be stopped if myositis develops, thus patients should be referred if they develop unusual muscle aches or pains. Statins should not be used in patients with liver disease. Simvastatin is taken at night and it is suggested that patients avoid grapefruit and follow a low-cholesterol diet.

18 E
From a communication standpoint this may mislead the patient around their prognosis.

19 A
Initial treatment of hypothyroidism with levothryoxine should be administered in lower doses for those aged over 50 years than for healthy, younger patients.

20 A
Avoid broad spectrum antibiotics due to increased risk of *C. difficile*, MRSA and resistant UTIs. See NICE guidance Antibiotic use: https://www.nice.org.uk/guidance/conditions-and-diseases/infections/antibiotic-use.

21 B
The overnight dexamethasone suppression test involves taking a dose of a corticosteroid medicine called dexamethasone to see how it affects the level of a hormone called cortisol in the blood. This test checks for Cushing's syndrome. In this condition, large

amounts of cortisol are produced by the adrenal glands. Source: http://www.homerton.nhs.uk/our-services/services-a-z/p/pathology/ information-for-healthcare-professionals/dynamic-function-testing/ dexamethasone-suppression-test-protocol/

22 C
Symptoms of tremor indicate salbutamol overuse and decreased peak expiratory flow indicates need for additional inhaled steroid.

23 B
Mild croup is usually self-limiting, but treatment with a single dose of a corticosteroid such as oral dexamethasone may be of benefit.

24 B
Treatment-resistant schizophrenia is diagnosed in individuals who do not respond to, or experience, serious side effects with at least two other antipsychotic medications. In these individuals clozapine is considered by NICE to be more effective at improving symptoms.

25 D
Tamoxifen should be taken daily not weekly. Tamoxifen may increase the risk of endometrial cancer with reports of irregular or unusual vaginal bleeding or discharge. It increases the efficacy of warfarin and therefore increases susceptibility to high INR readings. Tamoxifen increases the risk of venous thromboembolism and a swollen leg could suggest a deep vein thrombosis which requires urgent medical attention in a hospital.

26 C
Opioids reduce peristalsis, increase the anal sphincter tone and promote absorption of water from the large intestine; this leads to hard stools and constipation. Ispaghula husk, a bulk-forming laxative, can cause obstruction and increase the risk of faecal impaction in opioid-induced constipation especially if fluid intake is inadequate. Constipation from opioid use is best treated with a stimulant laxative, or a stool-softening laxative, or both if necessary. Adequate fluid intake should be maintained. Source MHRA: http://www.mhra.gov.uk/opioids-learning-module/con143740?use secondary=&showpage=6

ANSWERS

27 A

Hirsutism (male-pattern hair growth in women) is not associated with cervical cancer.

28 C

Furesomide is a loop diuretic that is strongly associated with urinary incontinence.

29 D

Risperidone causes parkinsonian side effects thus exacerbating the underlying disease.

30 B

Apixaban is licensed for the prophylaxis of stroke in patients with non-valvular AF and at least one risk factor such as previous stroke.

31 A

A baseline chest X-ray should be conducted due to the risk of pulmonary toxicity. Liver function should be monitored throughout therapy and not only in cases of suspected hepatotoxicity. Renal failure is not a side effect of amiodarone and creatinine levels are not used to determine the dose of amiodarone. Corneal microdeposits are reversible.

32 B

A sore throat is a sign of infection which could be due to carbimazole-induced bone marrow suppression.

33 C

Initial dose of ramipril is subject to renal function and should be established at baseline. Reduced white blood cell count is a rare side effect of ACE inhibitors and thus is not necessary to measure at baseline.

34 E

Severe cases of hepatocellular injury have been reported with tolcapone. Potentially life-threatening hepatotoxicity including fulminant hepatitis reported rarely, usually in women and during the first 6 months, but late-onset liver injury also reported; test liver function before treatment, and monitor every 2 weeks for first year, every 4 weeks for next 6 months and then every 8 weeks thereafter (restart monitoring schedule if dose increased); discontinue if abnormal liver function tests or symptoms of liver disorder and do not re-introduce tolcapone once discontinued.

35 B
Prophylactic enoxaparin is contraindicated following an acute stroke (for at least two months but varies according to hospital).

36 B
Extravasation is an oncological emergency. It is the unintentional leakage of intravenous drugs into the surrounding perivascular tissue or subcutaneous spaces. Patient factors include age, as young and elderly patients tend to have small mobile veins with friable skin and patients with long-term side effects from treatment e.g. peripheral neuropathy. Statins do not affect extravasation rates. However, concurrent medication with analgesics, anticoagulants, anti-fibrinolytics, vasodilators, hormone therapy, steroids, diuretics, anti-histamines, intravenous antibiotics may, depending on the drug increase blood flow, predispose patients to bleeding, suppress the inflammatory response, reduce pain sensation etc. See: https://www.england.nhs.uk/mids-east/wp-content/uploads/sites/7/2018/04/management-extravasation-of-a-systemic-anti-cancer-therapy-including-cytotoxic-agents.pdf

37 C
Levothyroxine has a narrow therapeutic drug, thus small increases in dose can cause hyperthyroid side effects such as tremor, tachycardia, weight loss, insomnia and anxiety.

38 B
The patient is suffering from athlete's foot and salicylic acid 15–50% is used for treatment of warts and would not be the appropriate advice. Griseofulvin is not the first-line treatment for athlete's foot and can cause side effects such as headache, nausea, and numbness.

39 E
Without treatment the condition often spreads to multiple toenails. However, cure is not achieved in 20–40 % of patients, with relapse occurring in 20–25% of people. Even in those in whom it is

successful, nails may appear abnormal for over 12 months due to their slow growth. It is more common in patients with diabetes. Source: https://patient.info/doctor/fungal-nail-infections-pro#nav-6

40 C

The patient is suffering from a severe flare up of ulcerative colitis (more than eight bowel movements and blood in stools), therefore IV steroids and IV fluids are required. Antibiotics should only be used if evidence of fever or raised levels of inflammatory markers. The patient is dehydrated and IV fluids are required, however dextrose is not first-line and given the frequency of diarrhoea it would not be appropriate to give over a 24 hour period. See: https://academic.oup.com/ecco-jcc/article/11/7/769/2962457

ANSWERS

Extended matching
answers

SECTION A

1 C
Shortness of breath is a feature of anaemia and usually confirmed with a full blood count. The symptoms of jaundiced appearance suggests haemolytic anaemia. The patient has been prescribed co-beneldopa which is a combination of benserazide and levdopa. Levdopa is associated with haemolytic anaemia which can be life threatening and the BNF recommends haematological monitoring.

2 E
The symptoms are suggestive of neutropenia with pyrexia. Disturbances in the production of neutrophils can lead to an increased risk of life-threatening infection. Fever, lethargy and sore throat are features of blood dyscrasia confirmed by the full blood count. The most likely cause is azathioprine, an immunosuppressant drug prescribed for rheumatoid arthritis. The BNF suggests patients on azathioprine should undergo blood monitoring every week for the first month and patient should be counselled.

3 F
Thrombocytopenia is defined as a reduction in platelet count – valproates are a class of drug most commonly involved.

4 B
Mr Albedi has hyperkalaemia associated with ECG abnormalities. This indicates a potential lethal risk of cardiac abnormalities. Ramipril, an ACEI, has the potential to increase potassium and is a precipitant drug causing hyperkalaemia.

5 F
SSRIs are suspected drugs to cause hyponatremia within a month of starting treatment. Syndrome of inappropriate antidiuretic hormone secretion (SIADH) appears to be part of the mechanism of hyponatraemia with the SSRIs, and inhibition of serotonin reuptake may be associated with a central increase in antidiuretic hormone (ADH) release, and hence induction of SIADH. Symptoms tend to improve once the SSRI is discontinued.

6 E
Hypokalaemia potentiates the effect of digoxin which may further contribute to the risk of arrhythmias.

7 G
Prophylaxis of stroke and systemic embolism in patients with non-valvular atrial fibrillation and with at least one of the following risk factors: congestive heart failure, hypertension, previous stroke or transient ischaemic attack, age ≥75 years, or diabetes mellitus.

8 F
The recommended dose for the initial treatment of acute DVT or PE is 15 mg twice daily for the first three weeks followed by 20 mg once daily for the continued treatment and prevention of recurrent DVT and PE. Short duration of therapy (at least 3 months) should be considered in patients with DVT or PE provoked by major transient risk factors (i.e. recent major surgery or trauma).

9 D
Following initial treatment of acute DVT and pulmonary embolism, the usual dose of 20 mg once daily can be given, but manufacturer advises to consider reducing to 15 mg once daily if creatinine clearance 15–49 mL/minute, and the risk of bleeding outweighs the risk of recurrent DVT or pulmonary embolism.

10 A
Rivaroxaban is a direct oral anticoagulant (DOAC) licensed for the prevention of atherothrombotic events in adult patients after an acute coronary syndrome with elevated cardiac biomarkers. It can be taken in combination with aspirin alone or aspirin and clopidogrel.

11 G

See BNF, chapter 9, section 2.1 on information about acute porphyrias. BNF states that oral contraceptives are not safe to take. Also check www.drugs-porphyria.org for further information on porphyria safe drug list.

12 B

Answer can be deduced by eliminating phenytoin after referring to BNF section 9.2.1. Additional info: According to porphyria.eu: http://porphyria.eu/he/content/anticonvulsants, clonazepam is safe to use as an anti-epileptic drug; phenytoin should not be used.

13 D

Non-nucleoside reverse transcriptase inhibitors such as efavirenz are not safe to take for HIV patients.

14 H

Simvastatin should be avoided as congenital anomalies have been reported.

15 H

Muscle wasting is a classic side effect of statins, especially in elderly patients.

16 B

These side effects are red flags to look out for with this medication. Patients are at risk of developing agranulocytosis and should be referred to the doctor immediately.

17 D

18 G

19 F

20 H

21 B

See BNF, Prescribing in palliative care. IV dose is half the oral daily dose.

ANSWERS

22 A
See BNF, Prescribing in palliative care. BNF equivalent doses of opioid analgesics state that oral morphine is a 10th of the dose of oral codeine.

23 A
Maximum breakthrough pain dose is 1/6th of total daily dose.

24 C
Concurrent administration of theophylline and ciprofloxacin may lead to toxic increases in theophylline levels (CYP450 interaction).

25 F
Sildenafil may markedly increase the hypotensive effects of nitrates.

26 H
This is a potassium-sparing diuretic that can lead to hyperkalaemia if potassium levels are not controlled.

27 G
Simvastatin interacts with macrolides, however other antibiotics listed above are fine to use.

28 E
This is the first step for asthma management. Suspected symptoms include diurnal variation in symptoms (typically worse at night) and worsening of symptoms with exercise.

29 D
Corticosteroids improve air flow by reducing airway inflammation, decreasing rate of treatment failure and risk of relapse, therefore decreasing the length of hospital stays.

30 H
Available as *Spiriva*® hard capsules for *HandiHaler*®, *Spiriva Respimat*® (soft mist inhaler) or tiotropium with *Zonda*® inhaler.

SECTION B

1 C
Co-trimoxazole contains trimethoprim which can interact with potassium-sparing diuretics to cause hyperkalaemia. See BNF, Appendix 1 Interactions or "Common antibiotic taken with a diuretic linked to sudden death, *The Pharmaceutical Journal*, 14 February 2015, Vol 294, No 7849, online | DOI: 10.1211/PJ.2015 .20067792".

2 G
Meropenem is known to significantly deplete valproate levels. These are both commonly used medicines so pharmacists should be aware of this contraindication.

3 E
Pharmacists should be aware of the interaction between simvastatin and macrolide antibiotics.

4 D
Both of these medicines are commonly prescribed in the community and it is possible that tetracycylines may be co-prescribed for acne. Concomitant use is contraindicated in Stockley's Drug Interactions.

5 E
Both erythromycin and domperidone should be used with caution in patients with cardiac history and at risk of QT prolongation. Erythromycin also interacts with domperidone to make this effect more prominent.

6 F
Linezolid has MOAI properties and can increase systemic serotonin concentrations. Couple this with taking fluoxetine and some patients can develop serotonin toxicity (syndrome) due to the heightened levels of serotonin in their body.

7 H
The question describes a typical presentation of *C. difficile* infection secondary to hospitalisation and antibiotic use. The white cell count is significantly raised and his albumin levels are low, both indicating

ANSWERS

severe *C. difficile* infection. Therefore, oral vancomycin is the recommended treatment option. See BNF monograph for vancomycin and PHE information.

8 D

Tetracyclines can chelate with cations, such as calcium, and will do so in developing bones. These agents should be avoided in children less than 12 years of age unless absolutely necessary.

9 F

See BNF monograph for linezolid. Blood disorders are a well-known side effect of linezolid, especially when given for more than 2 weeks. White cell depletion and thrombocytopenia can occur with beta-lactam agents but this is uncommon and associated with long-term treatment.

10 C

While extremely rare, all medicines including antibiotics can cause Stevens-Johnson syndrome and toxic epidermal necrolysis. Co-trimoxazole is more commonly implicated with this condition and pharmacists should be aware of this risk. More information can be found from the EuroSCAR study and the Clinical Pharmacist article covering this topic.

11 H

See BNF monograph for spironolactone, which discusses the use of high dose spironolactone in ascites secondary to liver cirrhosis.

12 B

See BNF monograph for bendroflumethiazide. This drug is generally ineffective for reducing blood pressure when eGFR is below 30 mL/min, but will still cause adverse effects.

13 A

See BNF, chapter 2, section 4.1 for information on calcium-channel blockers and BNF monograph for amlodipine. Calcium channel blockers are commonly implicated in ankle swelling.

14 H
Spironolactone, due to its mode of action, is associated with the development of gynaecomastia in men, breast pain, and excessive hair growth.

15 E
See BNF introductory information to chapter 2, section 4.1 for information on hypertension in pregnancy. Labetalol generally used first-line, while methyldopa is an alternative.

16 A
The SGLT2 inhibitors reduce glucose resorption in the kidneys which leads to a higher glucose concentration in the urine. In turn this causes increased rates of UTI and vaginal thrush.

17 H
See BNF monograph for pioglitazone regarding risks of bladder cancer.

18 G
Patients with reduced renal function should avoid metformin as it can precipitate lactic acidosis. Heart failure can cause reduced renal perfusion and therefore reduced function.

19 G
Metformin increases insulin utilisation in peripheral tissues and can cause a reduction in weight. It can be added to insulin for type 1 diabetics if patients need large doses and are developing insulin resistance. See NICE guidance on type 1 diabetes adjunct treatment: https://www.nice.org.uk/guidance/ng17

20 H
See BNF monograph for pioglitazone. Pioglitazone should be used with caution in patients with cardiovascular disease and is contraindicated in patients with a history of heart failure. Liraglutide should be used with caution in people with mild congestive heart failure or left ventricular dysfunction; it is contraindicated in moderate to severe congestive heart failure.

ANSWERS

21 F

See BNF monograph for liraglutide and the SPC for *Saxenda®*, which is licensed as an adjunct for weight loss.

22 G

See BNF monograph for phenytoin regarding safety information for intravenous use of phenytoin, which warrants ECG and blood pressure monitoring.

23 H

See updated guidelines from the MHRA on the contraindication of sodium valproate in women of childbearing age not on a pregnancy prevention programme.

24 E

See BNF introductory information to chapter 4, section 2 for information on status epilepticus that advises on the use of IV lorazepam to stop convulsions lasting longer than 5 minutes.

25 A

See BNF monograph and SPC for clobazam. This is used as an adjunct to epilepsy management and is generally taken at night initially. It may be taken multiple times a day when doses increase above 30 mg.

26 G

See BNF monograph for phenytoin that discusses the issue of acne, and other facial problems, in adolescents taking phenytoin.

27 I

Sodium bicarbonate is alkaline and can relieve acidosis and restore the pH balance in the blood. It can be given intravenously in acute situations, although some kidney disease patients may take this orally long-term to prevent acidosis.

28 B

Calcium carbonate, and calcium acetate, along with other products can be used to reduce serum phosphate. They do this by binding to dietary phosphate and preventing its absorption.

29 G
Salbutamol drives potassium into cells, which is why it can be used in the treatment of hyperkalaemia.

30 C
Calcium gluconate protects the myocardium from the effects of high potassium, which can cause arrhythmias and fibrillation.

31 H
Carbamazepine and mirtazapine can cause hyponatraemia individually, so it would be expected to have an additive effect when these medicines are used concomitantly. Hyponatraemia is known to cause confusion and drowsiness.

32 F
See the Cochrane glossary – https://community.cochrane.org/glossary#letter-P

33 B
See the Cochrane glossary – https://community.cochrane.org/glossary#letter-C

34 D
See the Cochrane glossary - https://community.cochrane.org/glossary#letter-N

35 G
See the Cochrane glossary - https://community.cochrane.org/glossary#letter-R

36 E
See the Cochrane glossary - https://community.cochrane.org/glossary#letter-O

37 F
Higher doses of salbutamol are associated with fine tremor and tachycardia. Lower doses should avoid this. While ipratropium and tiotropium can cause tachycardia they are unlikely to cause fine tremor.

ANSWERS

38 H
See MHRA safety information for the prescribing of tiotropium dry powder inhalers, which discusses the risks of inhaling the capsule when switching between brands and not supporting patients with this change.

39 B
Carbocisteine takes days to weeks to reach full effect so it is not useful to give this acutely for short courses – NICE guidance recommends it should only be used in patients who require long term reduction in mucous viscosity: www.nice.org.uk/guidance/cg101.

40 B
Carbocisteine is a mucolytic and can reduce the viscosity of gastric mucous as well as respiratory mucous. This can increase the risk of peptic ulcers. Carbocisteine is contraindicated in active peptic ulceration. Steroids can increase risk of peptic ulceration, but this is not a contraindication.

SECTION C

1 G

Venlafaxine is not recommended as a first-line by NICE and is the only antidepressant listed that belongs to the SNRI class.

2 B

Buspirone is an anti-anxiety medicine which is prescribed for short periods of time to help ease symptoms of anxiety. The dose of 5 mg two to three times a day does not match any of the other listed medicines.

3 A

Neuropathic pain occurs as a result of damage to neural tissue and is generally managed with a tricyclic antidepressant or with certain antiepileptic drugs. Amitriptyline (unlicensed indication) is the first-line and most effective treatment for neuropathic pain. Amitriptyline hydrochloride can be used in combination with pregabalin if the patient has an inadequate response to either drug at the maximum tolerated dose.

4 E

Sertraline is safe post-myocardial infarction and considered the drug of choice in these patients. However, citalopram is associated with dose-dependent QT interval prolongation and is contraindicated in patients with known QT interval prolongation or congenital long QT syndrome.

5 H

Zopiclone is indicated for the short-term treatment of insomnia. A single course of treatment should not continue for longer than 4 weeks including any tapering off. Extension beyond the maximum treatment period should not take place without re-evaluation of the patient's status.

6 G

Molluscum contagiosum is a skin infection caused by the molluscum contagiosum virus and is common in children. Molluscum can be passed on by direct contact with a molluscum lesion on the skin of an infected person. The virus can also be spread through contact with contaminated objects, such as towels, clothing, or toys. Umbilicated papules have a central dell or dimple which is characteristic of molluscum.

7 D
Impetigo is a highly contagious, superficial skin infection that most commonly affects children two to five years of age.

8 B
Croup is one of the most common causes of upper airway obstruction in young children. It is characterised by sudden onset of barking cough, inspiratory stridor and respiratory distress caused by upper airway inflammation secondary to a viral infection. The clinical benefit of administering the corticosteroid dexamethasone in croup is well established and should be considered for treating all children presenting with croup and symptoms ranging from moderate to severe. Improvement generally begins within 2 to 3 hours after a single oral dose of dexamethasone and persists for 24 to 48 hours.

9 F
Clinical presentation of meningitis may include fever and headache, stiff neck (generally not present in children under the age of one year or in patients with altered mental state), back rigidity, bulging fontanelle (in infants), photophobia, Kernig's sign (pain and resistance on passive knee extension with hips fully flexed). Brudzinski's sign (hips flex on bending the head forward), paresis, focal neurological deficits (including cranial nerve involvement and abnormal pupils) and seizures. See full list of symptoms here: https://patient.info/doctor/meningitis-pro

10 E
Measles is a highly infectious illness that mainly affects children but can occur at any age. It is rare in the UK, due to immunisation. The illness is unpleasant but most children fully recover. However, some children develop serious complications. Children are usually quite unwell and miserable for 3–5 days. After this, the fever tends to ease and then the rash fades.

11 E
Ototoxicity has been observed in up to 31% of patients treated with a single dose of cisplatin 50 mg/m^2 and is manifested by

tinnitus and/or hearing loss in the frequency range (4000 to 8000 Hz). Cisplatin can also cause nephrotoxicity but as the question states that the toxicity is "manifested by tinnitus" this rules out nephrotoxicity.

12 A

Cardiotoxicity is a risk of anthracycline treatment that may be manifested by early (i.e. acute) or late (i.e. delayed) events.

13 G

Pulmonary toxicity caused by bleomycin is both dose-related and age-related. The earliest symptom associated with pulmonary toxicity of bleomycin is dyspnoea. Fine rales are the earliest sign. If pulmonary changes are noted, treatment should be discontinued until it can be determined if they are drug related.

14 C

Gentamicin can cause both ototoxicity and nephrotoxicity. However, as the patient is displaying signs of renal impairment and is also on an NSAID, in this case nephrotoxicity is more likely.

15 H

The patient is showing signs of toxic epidermal necrosis, a severe life-threatening bullous reaction. Amiodarone can also cause pulmonary toxicity, phototoxicity, and hepatoxicity, but these adverse effects were not demonstrated in the case.

16 F

Due to isotretinoin-induced photosensitivity, exposure to intense sunlight or to UV rays should be avoided. Where necessary, a sun-protection product with a high protection factor of at least SPF 15 should be used. Aggressive chemical dermabrasion and cutaneous laser treatment should be avoided in patients on isotretinoin for a period of 5–6 months after the end of the treatment because of the risk of hypertrophic scarring in atypical areas and more rarely post inflammatory hyper- or hypopigmentation in treated areas. Wax depilation should be avoided in patients on isotretinoin for at least a period of 6 months after treatment because of the risk of epidermal stripping.

ANSWERS

17 C
Amphotericin B is highly nephrotoxic and serum potassium and magnesium levels should be checked once weekly alongside renal, hepatic and haematopoietic function. While amphotericin B has other toxic effects, serum creatinine is a specific indicator of renal function.

18 A
Carbamazepine is first-line treatment for trigeminal neuralgia which is a chronic pain condition that affects the trigeminal nerves around the face. See SPC for *Tegretol*® tablets 100 mg.

19 A
See BNF monograph for carbamazepine.

20 C
See BNF monograph for lorazepam. The patient is suffering from status epilepticus. Note that while IV diazepam is effective in treating status epilepticus it also carries a high risk of thrombophlebitis which is reduced by using an emulsion formulation. Absorption of diazepam from intramuscular injection or from suppositories is too slow for treatment of status epilepticus.

21 F
See BNF monograph for sodium valproate.

22 F
See BNF monograph for sodium valproate.

23 F
See BNF monograph for sodium valproate and MHRA: https://www.gov.uk/government/news/valproate-banned-without-the-pregnancy-prevention-programme

24 A
BCG vaccine is given at birth only to babies at risk e.g. where TB is endemic.

25 B
See BNF, chapter 14, section 4. Cholera vaccine is an oral vaccine.

26 E
See BNF, chapter 14, section 4 and https://www.gov.uk/government/news/hpv-vaccine-to-be-given-to-boys-in-england.

27 G
See BNF, chapter 14, section 4.

28 E
There are two main types of cholesterol: low-density lipoprotein (LDL), or "bad" cholesterol, and high-density lipoprotein (HDL), or "good" cholesterol, which helps to reduce levels of LDL.

29 H
Hashimoto's disease can cause primary hypothyroidism with decreased levels of T4 causing a compensatory increase in levels of thyroid stimulating hormone (TSH). The TSH target range is approximately 0.5–5 mIU/L.

30 F
MCV stands for mean corpuscular volume. There are three main types of corpuscles in your blood – red blood cells, white blood cells and platelets. An MCV blood test measures the average size of red blood cells (erythrocytes). Microcytic red blood cells have a low MCV, and macrocytic red blood cells (high MCV) are usually indicative of megaloblastic anaemia and liver disease.

31 A
Assessing liver function markers such as bilirubin, alanine aminotransferase (ALT), the less commonly measured aspartate aminotransferase (AST) and alkaline phosphate (ALP) at elevated levels indicate hepatocyte injury or cholestasis.

32 B
Vancomycin is a nephrotoxic drug and causes hypoperfusion of the kidneys and is further exacerbated by dehydration. The kidneys maintain blood creatinine in a normal range. Creatinine has been found to be a fairly reliable indicator of kidney function. Elevated creatinine level signifies impaired kidney function.

33 A

Anti-progesterone mifepristone and the prostaglandin analogue are prescribed for termination of pregnancy.

34 C

This patient is suffering from endometriosis. Endometriosis is sometimes mistaken for other conditions that can cause pelvic pain, such as pelvic inflammatory disease (PID) or ovarian cysts. It may be confused with irritable bowel syndrome (IBS), a condition that causes bouts of diarrhoea, constipation and abdominal cramping. IBS can accompany endometriosis, which can complicate the diagnosis.

35 C

Although the exact cause of endometriosis is not certain, possible explanations include:

- Retrograde menstruation – In retrograde menstruation, menstrual blood containing endometrial cells flows back through the fallopian tubes and into the pelvic cavity instead of out of the body. These displaced endometrial cells stick to the pelvic walls and surfaces of pelvic organs, where they grow and continue to thicken and bleed over the course of each menstrual cycle.
- Transformation of peritoneal cells – In what's known as the 'induction theory', experts propose that hormones or immune factors promote transformation of peritoneal cells (cells that line the inner side of your abdomen) into endometrial cells.
- Embryonic cell transformation – Hormones such as oestrogen may transform embryonic cells (cells in the earliest stages of development) into endometrial cell implants during puberty.

36 G

Pre-eclampsia occurs only in pregnancy and is of unknown aetiology. Although rare, it is a significant cause of maternal and fetal morbidity and mortality. Pre-eclampsia is defined by the new onset of elevated blood pressure and proteinuria after 20 weeks of gestation. It is considered severe if blood pressure and proteinuria are increased substantially or symptoms of end-organ damage (including fetal growth restriction) occur. There is no single reliable, cost-effective screening test for pre-eclampsia, and there are no well-established measures for primary prevention. Management before the onset of labour includes close monitoring of maternal and fetal status. Management during delivery includes seizure prophylaxis with magnesium sulfate and, if necessary, medical management of hypertension. Delivery remains the ultimate treatment. Access to prenatal care, early detection of the disorder, careful monitoring, and appropriate management are crucial elements in the prevention of pre-eclampsia-related deaths. Source: https://www.aafp.org/afp/2004/1215/p2317.html.

37 F

Polycystic ovaries on ultrasound are very common and can be seen in up to 33% of women of reproductive age. However, the majority of women with polycystic ovaries do not have features of polycystic ovary syndrome (PCOS) and do not require intervention. Prevalence figures vary depending on diagnostic criteria used, but PCOS is thought to affect 5–15% of women of reproductive age. Metformin is sometimes prescribed off-license to treat this condition.

38 H

The symptoms indicate that the patient is suffering from trichomoniasis, a very common sexually transmitted disease (STD). It is caused by infection with a protozoan parasite called *trichomonas vaginalis*. About 70% of infected people do not have any signs or symptoms. It is treated with oral metronidazole 400–500 mg.

39 E

Pelvic inflammatory disease (PID) is a clinical syndrome that results from the ascension of microorganisms from the cervix and vagina to the upper genital tract. PID can lead to infertility and permanent damage of a woman's reproductive organs. PID is a serious complication of some STDs, especially chlamydia and gonorrhoea. May be treated with ceftriaxone 500 mg as a single intramuscular (IM) dose, followed by doxycycline 10 mg orally twice daily and metronidazole 400 mg twice daily for 14 days. Source: https://patient.info/doctor/pelvic-inflammatory-disease-pro#nav-4

40 B

Cigarette smoking, and more than three full-term pregnancies are all risk factors for cervical cancer. Therefore, this patient should undergo a cervical screening test.

SECTION D

1 B
   See Symptoms in the Pharmacy: A Guide to the Management of Common Illness, 6th Ed., Blenkinsopp, Paxton and Blenkinsopp. There is a sticky discharge so this indicates bacterial, not allergic, conjunctivitis.

2 C
   See Symptoms in the Pharmacy: A Guide to the Management of Common Illness, 6th Ed., Blenkinsopp, Paxton and Blenkinsopp. There is itching of the scalp and the white dots attached to the hair close to the scalp indicate louse eggs or nits.

3 D
   See Symptoms in the Pharmacy: A Guide to the Management of Common Illness, 6th Ed., Blenkinsopp, Paxton and Blenkinsopp. There are a number of sores in the mouth but no complaint of white plaques covering the tongue/mouth, hence not oral thrush. Minor aphthous ulcers usually occur in crops of one to five, with common sites being the tongue, inside the lips and cheeks.

4 E
   See Symptoms in the Pharmacy: A Guide to the Management of Common Illness, 6th Ed., Blenkinsopp, Paxton and Blenkinsopp. Oral thrush is common in babies and can affect the surface of the tongue and the inside of the cheeks – white patches known as plaques occur due to candida.

5 G
   See Symptoms in the Pharmacy: A Guide to the Management of Common Illness, 6th Ed., Blenkinsopp, Paxton and Blenkinsopp. High level use of swimming pools has contributed to high risk of verrucae – warts that appear on the sole of the foot are known as a verruca. The pressure from the body's weight pushes the lesion inwards and eventually produces pain when weight is applied during walking. The black dots are thrombosed capillaries which can indicate the presence of a verruca.

6 D

See MEP 42, Controlled drugs, Classification. A schedule 3 controlled drug prescription is valid for 28 days.

7 E

See MEP 42, Controlled drugs, Prescription requirements for schedule 2 and 3 controlled drugs. The Department of Health and Scottish Government have issued strong recommendations that the maximum quantity of schedule 2, 3 or 4 controlled drugs prescribed should not exceed 30 days.

8 E

See MEP 42, Professional and legal issues: prescription-only medicines, Exemptions: sale and supply without a prescription, Emergency supply. No more than 30 days can be supplied unless the POM is an inhaler, insulin, an ointment or a cream – the smallest pack size available should be supplied.

9 A

See MEP 42, Professional and legal issues: prescription-only medicines, Exemptions: sale and supply without a prescription, Emergency supply. The prescriber must agree to provide a written prescription within 72 hours.

10 F

See MEP 42, Professional and legal issues: prescription-only medicines, General prescription requirements. A private prescription is valid for up to 6 months from the appropriate date. For private prescriptions, the appropriate date will always be the date on which it was signed.

11 G

See BNF monograph for lansoprazole. All proton pump inhibitors have the potential to cause hyponatraemia.

12 A

See BNF monograph for empagliflozin for safety information about diabetic ketoacidosis with empagliflozin.

ANSWERS

13 F

See BNF information on loop diuretics. Furosemide can cause hypokalaemia, and hypokalaemia can predispose patients to digoxin toxicity – see BNF monograph for digoxin.

14 E

Symptoms described are of hypoglycaemia and sulphonylureas tend to cause this in elderly patients.

15 D

NSAIDs can increase blood pressure in patients with hypertension.

Calculations answers

SECTION A

1 37 kg/m^2
   1 foot = 304.8 mm and 1 inch = 25.4 mm therefore 4' 11'' = 1.498 m
   13 st = 82.55 kg and 1 lb = 0.45 kg, therefore 13 st 1 lb = 83 kg
   Thus, BMI (kg/m^2) = 83 ÷1.498^2 = 36.987 kg/m^2
   Note: calculating as 83 ÷ (1.50 × 1.50) will also give you 36.899 kg/m^2

2 29.1 kg
   Calculate target weight: (24 × 1.498) × 1.498 = 53.8561 kg
   Calculate weight to be lost: 83 − 53.8561 = 29.1439 kg

3 39.3 mL/min
   The SPC gives the following equation for adult males:
   eGFR = (Weight [kg] × 140 − age [years]) ÷ 72 × serum creatinine (mg/dl)
   Therefore, eGFR = (83 × 140 − 63) ÷ 72 × 2.26 = 6391 ÷ 162.72 = 39.2761

4 20 mg
   Patient is receiving 120 mg morphine each day
   Therefore, rescue dose: 120 ÷ 6 = 20 mg

5 23 mL
   SPC states 100 mg phenytoin sodium is molecularly equivalent to 92 mg phenytoin
   Therefore, patient needs 92 mg × 1.5 = 138 mg phenytoin as liquid per dose
   SPC states concentration is 30 mg/5 mL, therefore 6 mg/mL
   138 mg ÷ 6 mg/mL = 23 mL

6 29 tablets

See BNF, chapter 5, section 5.2 – *Malarone*® should be started 1–2 days before entering an endemic area and continued for a week after leaving. Patient at risk for the whole journey.

Minimum number of tablets would allow for 1 day before endemic area, not 2.

Therefore, Miss L should receive 29 tablets (1 + 21 + 7)

Candidates are encouraged to utilise the NaTHNaC website (https://travelhealthpro.org.uk/) when giving advice on travel health. This website also gives dosing guidance, but the BNF remains a useful reference for other medicine information.

7 1200 mg

Place the numbers you have been supplied into the equation given:

Total iron dose = $58 \times ([14 - 9] \times 2.4) + 500 = 1196$ mg

Note: If you add the constant (500) before multiplying by the body weight you will get this wrong.

8 3 vials

Number of vials = $(69 \times 3.7) \div 100 = 255.3 \div 100 = 2.553$ vials

Need to supply whole vials, so need to round up to 3.

9 50 mg

See BNFC, chapter 6, section 2 – Use the glucocorticoid conversion table

800 mcg methylprednisolone = 1 mg prednisolone

Thus: 8 mg methylprednisolone = 10 mg prednisolone

10 mg methylprednisolone = 12.5 mg prednisolone

Therefore, as going from QDS to OD, total dose = $4 \times 12.5 = 50$ mg prednisolone

10 112 tablets

40 mg daily = 8×5 mg tablets

8 tablets × 14 days = 112 tablets

11 19.87 mL

Molecular weight of potassium chloride (KCl) = $39 + 35.5 = 74.5$

Moles = mass ÷ molecular weight. Rearrange to give: mass = moles × molecular weight

Thus, mass needed per bag = 40 mmols × 74.5 = 2980 mg

Given 15% v/w vials = 15000 mg per 100 mL = 150 mg/mL = 1 mg in 0.00666 mL
Therefore: 0.00666 × 2980 = 19.8666 mL of KCl solution

12 5 g
Note: Need to use alligation method here, not as simple as adding assumed amount of solid.

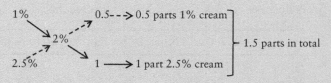

Need to make 15 g, so: 15 g ÷ 1.5 parts = 10 g per part
Therefore: 0.5 × 10 = 5 g of 1% cream

13 1579 mg
Alligation can be used here again.

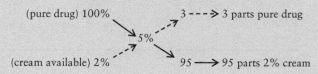

Thus: The 2% cream makes 95 parts of final 98 parts
As we only know the starting weight we work out parts from the original cream only
Therefore: 50 g ÷ 95 parts = 0.526 g/part
Therefore: 3 parts × 0.526 g/part = 1.579 g salicylic acid to add
Can check answer: ([1.00 + 1.58] ÷ [50 + 1.58]) × 100 = 5.00 %

14 2 bottles
Patient needs 5 mL per dose, therefore 20 mL per day
20 mL × 7 days = 140 mL
Bottles are 100 mL in size, so two bottles needed

15 7.1 mL/hour
Dose = 3 mcg × 63.2 kg = 189.6 mcg/minute
160 mg in 100 mL = 1.6 mg/mL = 1600 mcg/mL
Therefore 189.6 mcg/min ÷ 1600 mcg/mL = 0.1185 mL/min
Thus, 0.1185 mL/min × 60 minutes = 7.11 mL/hour

16 560 ampoules
Each dose needs 4 ampoules (2 per 1 g flucloxacillin, with each dose needing two 1 g vials)
Therefore patient requires 16 ampoules per day
$16 \times (5 \times 7) = 560$ ampoules

17 455 tablets
Generally easier to draw up a table to calculate the dose

Dose	No. days	No. tabs per day	Total no. tabs
50 mg	14	10	140
45 mg	7	9	63
40 mg	7	8	56
35 mg	7	7	49
30 mg	7	6	42
25 mg	7	5	35
20 mg	7	4	28
15 mg	7	3	21
10 mg	7	2	14
5 mg	7	1	7
Total			455

18 336 tablets
Need 2 tablets per dose ($2 \times 480 = 960$), which is equivalent to 4 tablets per dosing day ($2 \times$ BD)
Only takes these three times a week, therefore will need $4 \times 3 = 12$ tablets per week
Thus, need to supply $12 \times 28 = 336$ tablets for the 28-week period

19 1500 mg
IBW $= 50 + (2.3 \times 9) = 70.7$ kg
Adjusted body weight $=$ IBW $+ (0.4 \times$ [ActBW $-$ IBW]) $= 70.7 + (0.4 \times [146 - 70.7]) = 100.82$ kg
Daily dose $= 100.82$ kg $\times 15$ mg/kg $= 1512.3$ mg
Note the answer is 1500 mg (i.e. three 400 mg tablets and three 100 mg tablets) as the monographs says to the nearest whole tablet and the smallest tablet comes in 100 mg strength

20 195 mcg
Pharmacists should know what each part of the equations mean and how to rearrange the equations
C_{pss} = Plasma concentration at steady state, F = bioavailability, D = dose, DigCl = Digoxin clearance, t = time interval between doses, and IBW = ideal body weight.

IBW = 50.0 + (2.3 × 10) = 73.0 kg
DigCl = (0.053 × 48.52) + (0.02 × 73) = 4.0316 L/hr
Need to rearrange C_{pss} equation to find D. Also, F becomes 1 (due to 100% bioavailable IV)
Thus: $D = (C_{pss} \times [DigCl \times t]) \div F = (2.0 \times [4.0316 \times 24]) \div 1 = 193.5168$ mcg
Revision on pharmacokinetics can be found in the PJ article Back to basics: pharmacokinetics: http://bit.ly/PJbasicPK

21 17 mL
Patient is taking 30 mg citalopram per day
Section 4.2 of the SPC gives conversion
30 mg citalopram tablets = 12 oral drops
Can derive that each drop contains 2 mg of citalopram. Therefore, if concentration is 40 mg/mL, each mL contains 20 drops
If taking 12 drops per day, will need 12 × 28 = 336 drops for supply
Thus, 336 drops ÷ 20 drops/mL = 16.8 mL
To whole number = 17 mL

22 45.36 mg
1200 tablets per hour over six hours = 1200 × 6 = 7200 tablets during the production
Each tablet has 6 mcg of coating. Therefore 7200 × 6 = 43,200 mcg = 43.2 mg
5% excess = 43.2 × 1.05 = 45.36 mg

23 5.98 g
Total mass need to be made is 6 × 1 g (6 supps, 6000 mg)
Displacement by morphine = 6 × 5 mg ÷ 1.6 = 18.75 mg
Therefore, mass of base (*Witepsol®*) = 6000 mg − 18.75 mg = 5981.25 mg = 5.98 g

24 8 mg patch
First work out A:
50 mg three times a day = 50 × 3 = 150 mg

100 mg MR at night $= 100 \times 0.7 = 70$ mg
A $= 220$ mg
Then work out B:
350 micrograms (0.35 mg) three times a day $= (0.35 \times 3) \times 100 =$
105 mg
B $= 105$ mg
LEDD $= (220 + 105) \times 0.55 = 178.75$ mg
Rotigotine dose $= 178.72 \div 20 = 8.9375$ mg
Prescribing information says to round to nearest 2 mg, therefore
8 mg closer than 10 mg

25 42 tablets
14 days at 2 mg $= 14 \times 2 \times 1 = 28$ tablets
14 days at 1 mg $= 14 \times 1 = 14$ tablets

26 77 mg
BSA $= \sqrt{([162 \times 82] \div 3600)} = \sqrt{3.69} = 1.9209$ m^2
Dose $= 40$ mg/m$^2 \times 1.9209$ m$^2 = 76.8375$ mg

27 £7645 GBP per 100 patients
Cost per 500 mg vial $= £76.90 \div 10 = £7.69$
Cost per 1 g vial $= £153.50 \div 10 = £15.35$
Current cost per patient $= £15.35 \times 3 \times 5 = £230.25$
New cost per patient $= £7.69 \times 4 \times 5 = £153.80$
Cost difference per patient $= £230.25 - £153.80 = £76.45$
Cost difference per 100 patients $= 76.45 \times 100 = £7645$

28 23.14 mg in 5 mL
First allocate the values for the equation
$f = 0.577$ (remove the minus to convert from freezing point to
freezing point depression)
$a = 0.3105$ (convert the 1% solution to the desired 2.5 % solution:
$2.5 \times 0.1242 = 0.3105$)
$b = 0.576$ (sodium chloride is the adjusting compound)

Perform the calculation:
$W = (0.577 - 0.3105) \div 0.576 = 0.2665 \div 0.576 = 0.4627\%$ w/v
0.4627% w/v $= 0.4627$ g in 100 mL $= 0.04627$ g in 10 mL $=$
46.27 mg in 10 mL
Therefore 23.135 mg sodium chloride in 5 mL product

29 58 units

First calculate how much alcohol per night: 11% of 750 mL wine = 82.5 mL alcohol

Then calculate units per night. If 10 mL alcohol = 1 unit, then 82.5 mL alcohol = 8.25 units

Finally, calculate weekly intake: 8.25 units × 7 nights = 57.75 units

30 47 mL

Need to use C1V1=C2V2. Can convert vols to % using the information given

If 30 vols = 9%, then 10 vols = 3%

Therefore 9% × V1 = 3% × 5 mL = 1.6667 mL of 30 vol solution per dose

Or seeing there is a three-fold difference between concentrations, can assume three-fold difference in quantity required: 5 mL ÷ 3 = 1.6667 mL

Thus, 1.6667 mL × 2 (doses per day) × 14 (days) = 46.6676 mL

SECTION B

1 0.5 mL
   Adrenaline (EpiPen) is available as a 1 in 1000 concentration
   1 in 1000 = 1 g in 1000 mL
   = 1000 mg ÷ 1000 mL = 1 mg/mL
   = 0.5 mg/0.5 mL

2 3
   ARR = EER − CER
   = 0.67 − 0.30
   = 0.37
   NNT = 1 ÷ 0.37 = 2.70 = 3

3 40 mg
   50 mg/5 mL = 10 mg/1 mL
   4 mL × 10 mg/mL = 40 mg
   Weight and age are not relevant to this question

4 18 mL
   Hydralazine ampoule = 20 mg/2 mL
   Adding 18 mL of NaCl 0.9% gives 1 mg/mL

5 4.69 mcg/mL
   1200 ÷ 60 = 20 hours

Time	Serum concentration
0 hrs	75 mcg/mL
5 hrs	37.5 mcg/mL
10 hrs	18.75 mc/mL
15 hrs	9.375 mcg/mL
20 hrs	4.69 mcg/mL

6 4 mL
   50 (kg) × 2 (mg/kg) = 100 mg
   50 mg in 2 mL
   100 mg in X mL

   X × 50 = 200
   X = 200 ÷ 50
   X = 4 mL

7 £18, 288
£24.99 − £9.75 = £15.24
£15.24 × 100 patients × 12 months = £18, 288

8 18 mL
Calculate total morphine oral dose in 24 hours
60 mg × 2 = 120 mg daily oral dose
Bioavailability: 0.3 therefore 120 mg × 0.3 = 36 mg of IV injection needed
Calculate how much 0.2% w/v solution for infusion is needed to give 36 mg
0.2% w/v = 0.2 g/100 mL
= 200 mg/100 mL
= 36 mg ÷ X mL
X = (36 × 100) ÷ 200 = 18 mL

9 10, 500 units
150 units × 70 kg = 10,500 units

10 100 mg
2.5 mL = 50 mg
2.5 mL = 50mg (first dose) + 2.5 mL = 50 mg (second dose) = 100 mg

11 200 mL
20 mg/kg = 20 mg × 40 kg = 800 mg per day
Calculate amount of syrup needed for each day:
100 mg/5 mL therefore (800 mg × 5 mL)/100 mg = 40 mL per dose
40 mL × 5 days = 200 mL

12 224 mL
500 mcg × 8 kg = 4000 mcg = 4 mg daily
Syrup available contains 50 mg/100 mL
50 mg =100 mL
5 mg =10 mL
4 mg = X mL
X = 40/5 = 8 mL
8 mL × 28 days = 224 mL

13 111 mL/hour
180 kcal per 100 mL therefore 2000 kcal in 1111.1 mL
1111.1 mL in 10 hours = 111.11 mL/hour

14 470 tablets
60 mg (12 tablets) daily for 10 days = 120 tablets
55 mg (11 tablets) daily for 7 days = 77 tablets
50 mg (10 tablets) daily for 7 days = 70 tablets
45 mg (9 tablets) daily for 7 days = 63 tablets
40 mg (8 tablets) daily for 7 days = 56 tablets
35 mg (7 tablets) daily for 7 days = 49 tablets
30 mg (6 tablets) daily for 7 days = 42 tablets
25 mg (5 tablets) daily for 7 days = 35 tablets
20 mg (4 tablets) daily for 7 days = 28 tablets
15 mg (3 tablets) daily for 7 days = 21 tablets
10 mg (2 tablets) daily for 7 days =14 tablets
5 mg (1 tablet) daily for 7 days = 7 tablets
Total needed = 582, you supply 112 and therefore still owe 470 tablets

15 184,000 units
Two batches of 10 plus extra 15% = $(10 \times 2) \times 1.15 = 23$ amps
Each amp = 2 mL. Therefore 23 amps = 46 mL
2000 units/0. 5 mL = 184,000 units

16 £1,707
Seretide®:
The difference in cost between the 250 and 125 Evohaler = £59.48 − £35.00 = £24.48
For 12 patients the savings would be £24.48 × 12 = £293.76
For 4 months this would be £293.76 × 4 = £1,175.04
Symbicort®:
The 400/12 inhalers last only for 1 month whereas the 200/6 inhalers last for 2 months, halving the costs. This means each patient switched would save £19
For 7 patients this would save £19 × 7 = £133
For 4 months this would be £133 × 4 = £532
Total savings = £532 + £1,175 = £1,707

17 298 g
1 mole of potassium chloride weighs 74.5 g (39 + 35.5)
1 mmol = 74.5 mg (divide both sides by 1,000)
The solution to be prepared contains 16 mmol potassium ions in 20 mL = 8 mmol in 10 mL
= 4,000 mmol in 5000 mL (8 mmol × 500)
Mass (g) = M_r × Moles = 74.5 mg × 4 mol = 298 g

18 6300 units

8 am to 5 pm = 9 hours

Rate = 1.75 mL per hour, therefore = 9 hrs × 1.75 mL = 15.75 mL

Heparin = 25,000 units in 50 mL

X units in 15.75 mL

$X \text{ units} = \frac{15.75 \text{ mL} \times 20,000 \text{ units}}{50 \text{ mL}} = 6300 \text{ units}$

19 1.2 mcg/L

First work out creatinine clearance

CrCl = ([140 – 73 yrs] × 70 kg × 1.04) ÷ 90 µmol/L = 54.2 mL/min

Then work out digoxin clearance

DigCl = (0.06 × 54.2 mL/min) + (0.05 × 70 kg) = 6.752 L/hr

Then plug numbers into C_{pss} equation

Note F = 1 for IV, D = dose, t = time interval in hours

C_{pss} = (1 × 187.5mcg) ÷ (6.752 L/hr × 24 hrs) = 1.16 mcg/L

To nearest decimal place = 1.2 mcg/L

20 57 g

DV = 0.6 meaning 0.6 g of menthol displaces 1 g of base (theobroma oil)

40 suppositories will weigh 62 g (40 × 1.55)

= 40 × 75 mg menthol = 3000 mg menthol or 3 g

If 0.6 g displaces 1 g of base, 3 g of base displaces = 3 ÷ 0.6 = 5 g

62 g − 5 g = 57 g base needed

SECTION C

1 4.5 mL
Step 1: Calculate how many mg per mL
100 mg in 5 mL therefore 20 mg in 1 mL
Hence 10 mg in 0.5 mL
Step 2: Calculate how many mL per 90 mg
0.5 mL × 9 = 90 mg in 4.5 mL

2 7.5 g
Step 1: Calculate daily dose
Each day the patient takes 3 × 500 mg = 1500 mg amoxicillin
Step 2: Calculate total for 5 days
5 × 1500 mg = 7500 mg
Step 3: Convert mg to g
7500 mg ÷ 1000 = 7.5g

3 129.3%
Step 1: Calculate the total amount of sodium taken daily
Each tablet contains 388 mg of sodium
388 mg × 8 tablets = 3104 mg = 3.104 g per day
Step 2: Calculate the daily dose as a percentage of daily allowance
of sodium
100% daily allowance = 2.4 g of sodium each day
3.104 ÷ 2.4 × 100 = 129.33%

4 2.07 g in 24 hours
Step 1: Calculate estimated creatinine clearance using the formula
provided

$$CrCl = \frac{(140 - 59) \times 69 \times 1.04}{275 \text{ (micromol/litre)}}$$

= 21.136 mL/min
Step 2: Read off dose adjustment from table and calculate
Therefore patient needs to take 15 mg/kg every 12 hours
15 mg × 69 kg = 1035 mg every 12 hours
Total over 24 hours = 2070 mg daily dose
Step 3: Convert into grams
In mg = 2.07g in 24 hours

5 300 mg daily
  Step 1: Calculate bioavailable dose received by oral suspension
  $200 \times 0.6 = 120$ mg BD
  Step 2: Calculate the equivalent total dose in oral tablets
  $120 \div 0.8 = 150$ mg BD
  Step 3: Calculate total daily dose
  150 mg $\times$ 2 = 300 mg daily

6 19 mL
  Step 1: Calculate total concentrate needed per dose i.e. 50 mg
  $4\% = 4$ g in 100 mL
  4000 mg in 100 mL
  100 mg in 2.5 mL
  50 mg in 1.25 mL
  Step 2: Calculate how many mL needed to cover 5 days
  1.25 mL $\times$ 3 = 3.75 mL per day
  3.75 mL $\times$ 5 = 18.75 mL
  19 mL to nearest whole mL

7 56 tablets
  Method 1:
  21 days' supply, so patient will have:
  Day 1 – 6 $\times$ 1 mg tablets = 6 tablets
  20 days doses remaining – 3 mg and 2 mg on alternate days therefore
  10 days – 2 $\times$ 1 mg tablets = 20 tablets
  10 days – 3 $\times$ 1 mg tablets = 30 tablets
  Total = 6 + 20 + 30 = 56 tabs
  Method 2:
  List the days
  6 for day 1
  3 for day 2
  2 for day 3
  3 for day 4
  2 for day 5
  3 for day 6
  2 for day 7
  3 for day 8
  2 for day 9
  3 for day 10
  2 for day 11
  3 for day 12
  2 for day 13

ANSWERS

3 for day 14
2 for day 15
3 for day 16
2 for day 17
3 for day 18
2 for day 19
3 for day 20
2 for day 21
$6 \times 1 = 6$
$3 \times 10 = 30$
$2 \times 10 = 20$
$6 + 30 + 20 = 56$ tablets of 1 mg warfarin

8 308 tablets
40 mg daily for 14 days = $8 \times 14 = 112$
35mg daily for 7 days = $7 \times 7 = 49$
30 mg daily for 7 days = $6 \times 7 = 42$
25 mg daily for 7 days = $5 \times 7 = 35$
20 mg daily for 7 days = $4 \times 7 = 28$
15 mg daily for 7 days = $3 \times 7 = 21$
10 mg daily for 7 days = $2 \times 7 = 14$
5 mg daily for 7 days = $1 \times 7 = 7$
$112 + 49 + 42 + 35 + 28 + 21 + 14 + 7 = 308$ tablets to be issued

9 2 bottles
Step 1: Calculate sprays to cover first 14 days
Dose = 2 sprays each nostril OD for 2/52 = 4 doses daily $\times$ 14 days
= 56 sprays
Step 2: Calculate number of sprays needed for the rest of the 6 weeks
1 spray per nostril OD for 6/52 = 2 doses daily $\times$ 42 days = 84
sprays
Step 3: Calculate total sprays needed for the 8 weeks
Total 56 + 84 = 140 sprays
Step 4: Calculate how many nasal sprays needed to cover 140 sprays
Each nasal spray contains 120 doses, therefore need 2 sprays needed
to cover 8 weeks in total

10 168 capsules
Step 1: Calculate daily dose of carbocisteine
250 mg/5 mL – patient takes 15 mL TDS
Step 2: Calculate the equivalent number of capsules per dose

Therefore 250 × 3 = 750 mg per dose
Each capsule has 375 mg therefore the patient takes 2 capsules per dose
Step 3: Calculate how many doses over 28 days
2 capsules TDS = 6 capsules taken daily
Over 28 days = 168 capsules

11 330 minutes
Method 1:
Step 1: Calculate amount of diamorphine to be administered-
We have 3 micrograms/mL therefore 30 micrograms in 10 mL
Step 2: Calculate the mL in syringe delivered
60 mL in 200 mm
10 mL in 33.33 mm
Step 3: Calculate rate of delivery
6 mm delivered in 60 mins
3.33 mm in 33 mins × 10 = 330 mins
Method 2:
Step 1: Calculate how many mL/mm in the syringe
60 mL in 20 cm = 60 mL in 200 mm
60 ÷ 200 = 0.3 mL/mm
Step 2: Calculate how many mL patient receives per hour
6 mm/hour therefore 0.3 mL × 6 = 1.8 mL per hour
Step 3: Calculate how long it takes to receive 30 micrograms diamorphine
We have a solution of 3 mcg/mL, so 30 micrograms in 10 mL
10 mL will be administered in 10 ÷ 1.8 = 5.5555555 hours
Step 4: Convert time of delivery from hours into minutes
5.55555 × 60 = 333.333333 minutes
330 mins to nearest ten minutes

12 24 g
Step 1: Calculate how much calamine in 4% cream
4% = 4 g in 100 g
Step 2: Calculate amount in 600 g
4 × 6 = 24 g

13 0.005% w/v
Step 1: Calculate how much hydrocortisone in milligrams is in 100 mL
350 mg in 7000 mL

50 mg in 1000 mL
5 mg in 100 mL
Step 2: Convert this to grams per 100 mL
5 mg ÷ 1000 = 0.005%

14 57.5 mL
Step 1: Calculate how much phenol needed in 100 mL
23% v/v = 23 mL in 100 mL
Step 2: Calculate how much phenol needed for 250 mL solution
250 ml is 2.5 times larger than 100 mL
23 mL × 2.5 = 57.5 mL

15 30
Step 1: Calculate the percentages involved

Drug given	Survived	Died
LowBeePee	230 (76.6666%)	70 (23.3333%)
Placebo	80 (80%)	20 (20%)

Step 2: Calculate ARR
80 − 76.66666 = 3.333333%
Step 3: Calculate NNT
100 ÷ 3.333333 = 30
i.e. 30 people would need to be treated with the drug in order for one patient to show beneficial effect from the drug

16 £51
Step 1: Calculate the cost of drugs including 20%

Drug	Cost price	Price to pay including 20% (multiply by 1.2)
Docusate capsules 100	£6.84/100 capsules	£8.21
Tramadol M/R 50 mg capsules	£16.83/60 capsules	£20.20
Nitromin (glyceryl trinitrate)	£4.49/180 dose bottle	£5.63
Total cost of drugs		£34.04

Step 2: Calculate dispensing fee
3 items = 3 × £4.50 = £13.50
Step 3: Add in a charge for a CD as tramadol is covered by this
Add £3.50
Step 4: Add all costs together including dispensing fee
£34.04 + £13.50 + £3.50 = £51.04
= £51 to nearest whole GBP

17   22.0 g
Step 1: Calculate the total weight of the 12 suppositories
12 × 2 = 24 g
Step 2: Calculate weight of paracetamol in the suppositories
250 mg × 12 = 3000 mg = 3 g
Step 3: Calculate effect of DV
If the DV is 1.5, this means that 1.5 g of paracetamol will displace
1 g of theobroma oil
Therefore 3 g of paracetamol will displace 2 g of theobroma oil
Step 4: Calculate weight of theobroma oil needed
Total weight of theobroma needed is 24 − 2 = 22 g

18   7.4 g
Step 1: Calculate the total weight of the 6 suppositories
6 × 1.5 g = 9 g
Step 2: Calculate weight of aspirin in the suppositories
300 mg × 6 = 1800 mg = 1.8 g
Step 3: Calculate effect of DV
If the DV is 1.1, this means that 1.1 g of aspirin will displace 1 g of
cocoa butter base
Therefore 1.8 g of aspirin will displace
(1 ÷ 1.1) × 1.8 = 1.636 g of cocoa butter base
Step 4: Calculate weight of cocoa butter needed
Total weight cocoa butter needed is 9 − 1.636 = 7.364 g

19   40.3 g
Step 1: Calculate the total weight of the 21 suppositories
21 × 2 g = 42 g
Step 2: Calculate weight of copper sulfate in the suppositories
250 mg × 21 = 5250 mg = 5.25 g
Step 3: Calculate effect of DV

ANSWERS

If the DV is 3, this means that 3 g of copper sulfate will displace 1 g of *Witepsol*® base
Therefore 5.25 g of copper sulfate will displace
$(1 \div 3) \times 5.25 = 1.75$ g of base
Step 4: Calculate weight of base needed
Total weight base needed is $42 - 1.75 = 40.25$ g

20 385 mmol
Step 1: Calculate how many milligrams of NaCl in 2500 mL
0.9% w/v = 0.9 g in 100 mL = 9 g in 1000 mL = 22.5 g in 2500 mL = 22500 mg in 2500 mL
Step 2: Calculate how much 1 mmol of NaCl weighs
1 mol of NaCl = 58.5 g
1 mmol of NaCl = 58.5 mg
1 mg = $1 \div 58.5 = 0.017$ mmol
22500 mg = 22500 mg $\times 0.017 = 384.615$ mmol

21 12.3 mL
Step 1: Calculate how many mmol in 2500 mL
We need 8 mmol/L i.e. 8 mmol per 1000 mL
Therefore 20 mmol per 2500 mL
Step 2: Calculate weight of magnesium needed for 2500 mL
1 mol = 246.5 g
1 mmol = 246.5 mg
20 mmol = 4930 mg = 4.93 g needed for 2500 mL
Step 3: Calculate how much magnesium sulphate 40% needed to give 4.93 g of drug
40% = 40 g/100 mL = 1 g per 2.5 ml
Therefore 4.93 g $\times$ 2.5 mL = 12.325 mL of magnesium 40% needed

22 22.05 g
Step 1: Calculate the weight of sodium bicarbonate in 1 mmol
1 mol = 84 g
1 mmol = 84 mg
Step 2: Calculate how many mmol of sodium bicarbonate in 1500 mL
175 mmol/L therefore 262.5 mmol in 1500 mL
Step 3: Calculate weight of 262.5 mmol
1 mmol = 84 mg
262.5 mmol = 22050 mg
Convert into grams 22.05 g

23 35.4 mg/L
Step 1: Add all information into the formula
Adjusted phenytoin mg/L $= \frac{21 \ (mg/L)}{(0.9 \times 23 \ [g/L]/42)+0.1}$
$= 35.42168674$ mg/L
Step 2: Round to one decimal place

24 3.67 mL/min
Step 1: Consider what the maximum rate is
Dose given over 30 minutes
Step 2: Calculate the volume needed to be administered
Total volume is 10 mL vial + 100 mL saline = 110 mL
Step 3: Calculate the rate in mL/min if 110 mL given over 30 mins
110mL ÷ 30 min = 3.6666mL/min
Step 4: Give answer to 2 decimal places

25 2.08 mm/hr
Method 1:
Step 1: Calculate total mm in the syringe
50 mm delivered over 24 hours
Step 2: Calculate how many mm delivered in an hour
50mm ÷ 24 hours = 2.083mm/hr
Method 2:
Step 1: Calculate the dose per hour
150 mg per 24 hours therefore
150 ÷ 24 = 6.25 mg/hour
Step 2: Calculate the concentration of cyclizine per mm in the syringe
driver to give 6.25 mg
150 mg in 5 cm
150 mg in 50 mm
6.25 mg in X mm
$X = (6.25 \div 150) \times 50 = 2.08333$ mm
Step 3: Round answer to 2 decimal places

26 9.4 mL/hour
Step 1: Calculate amount needed by patient
2.75 mcg/kg/min
$2.75 \times 71 = 195.25$ mcg/min
Step 2: Calculate how many micrograms per mL in the dopamine
infusion
Infusion bag has 125 mg = 125,000 mcg in 100 mL
Therefore 1250 mcg per 1 mL

Step 3: Calculate how many mL of infusion contains 195.25 mcg
195.25 ÷ 1250 = 0.1562 mL/min
Step 4: Calculate how many mL/hour
0.1562 mL × 60 = 9.372 mL/hour

27 0.72 mL
Step 1: Calculate daily dose
40 mg OD
Step 2: Calculate the equivalent dose from oral to injection
40 × 0.9 = 36 mg daily by injection
Step 3: Calculate how much 5% solution needed
We have 5% solution
5 g/100 mL
5,000 mg/100 mL
50 mg/1 mL
1 mg in 0.02 mL
Step 3: Calculate how many mLs give 36 mg
0.02 mL × 36 = 0.72 mL
= 0.72 mL

28 14.14 g
Step 1: Use alligation method to calculate amount of parts in total

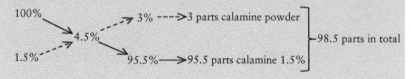

Step 2: Calculate how much one part weighs
We are adding the powder to 450 g so 450 g ÷ 95.5 parts = 4.7120418 g/part
Step 3: Calculate how much 3 parts weigh
Therefore 4.71 g/part × 3 parts = 14.13612 g

29 49 drops per minute
Step 1: Calculate the dose
Dose = 500 × 73 = 36,500 mcg/hour
Step 2: Calculate dose per minute
36500 ÷ 60 = 608.333 mcg/minute

Step 3: Calculate amount of preparation needed per minute
= 25 mg/100 mL
= 0.25 mg/1 mL
= 250 mcg/mL
We need 608.333 mcg
608 ÷ 250 = 2.43333 mL/minute
Step 4: Calculate how many drops in 2.43 mL
0.05 mL = 1 drop
2.433333 ÷ 0.05mL = 48.66 drops/minute
= 49 drops/minute

30 138 minutes
Step 1: Calculate total amount of drug in the infusion
Dose = 0.3/kg = 0.3 g × 15 = 4.5 g given in total in the infusion
Step 2: Calculate how much 10% solution is required to give 4.5 g
10% solution = 10 g per 100 mL = 0.1 g/1 mL
4.5 g ÷ 0.1 g/mL = 45 mL in total to be given
Step 3: Calculate infusion rate and how much infusion remains
0.75 mL × 15 × 0.75 hour = 8.4375 mL
1.2 mL × 15 × 0.5 hour = 9 mL
Total of first two parts of infusion: 9 + 8.4375 mL = 17.4375
Remainder of infusion: 45 mL – 17.44 mL = 27.56 mL
Step 4: Calculate how long the remainder of infusion will be given
in minutes
1.75 mL × 15 × Y hours = 27.56 mL
Y hours = 27.56 ÷ 26.25 = 1.0499 hours
1.0499 × 60 = 62.99 minutes
Step 5: Add up how long each infusion takes place for
Total = 45 minutes + 30 minutes + 62.99 = 137.99 minutes
= 138 minutes

31 125 mL
Step 1: Calculate dose needed by child
Dose = 2 mg/kg therefore 22 kg × 2 mg = 44 mg
44 mg daily
Step 2: Calculate how much suspension is needed to give 44 mg
50 mg/5 mL suspension
= 10 mg/mL
Therefore we need to multiply by 4.4 to get 44 mg
1 × 4.4 = 4.4 mL daily

Step 3: Calculate 28 days' supply
4.4 mL × 28 = 123.2 mL
Step 4: Round up to nearest 5 mL
= 125 mL

32 24 capsules
Step 1: Calculate dose needed at 30 mg/m^2
SM = 1.33 m^2, so 30 × 1.33 = 39.9 mg daily
Step 2: Calculate the number of capsules needed per day
39.9 ÷ 5 mg = 7.98 capsules each day
Closest amount per day = 8 capsules
Step 3: Calculate number of capsules for 3 days
8 × 3 days = 24 capsules

33 11.41 g
Step 1: Calculate how much 1 millimole of morphine weighs
1 mole of morphine = 285.3 g
1 mmol = 285.3 mg
Step 2: Calculate the weight of 40 millimoles
40 × 258.3 = 11,412 mg
Step 3: Convert into grams
11412 ÷ 1000 = 11.412 g

34 4 tablets
Step 1: Calculate total amount calcium taken each day from *Accrete*®
tablets
Convert *Accrete*® 1 TDS
600 mg × 3 = 1800 mg calcium daily
Step 2: Calculate total number of *Calceos*® tablets needed to give
1800 mg
1800 mg ÷ 500 = 3.6 tablets daily
Step 3: Calculate total tablets daily to nearest whole tablet
4 tablets daily for equivalent dose

35 140 mL
Step 1: Calculate quantity of solution needed to give 5 mg
500 mcg/1 mL = 0.5 mg per 1 mL
0.5 mg × 10 = 5 mg per 10 mL therefore PR needs 10 mL daily
Step 2: Calculate the quantity needed to cover 14 days
10 × 14 = 140 mL

36 29 mL/hr
Step 1: Calculate dose per hour
Dose = 0.1 g × 58 = 5.8 g per hour

Step 2: Calculate how many mL of infusion gives 5.8 g
Infusion = 150,000 mg per 750 mL
= 150 g per 750 mL
= 1 g per 5 mL
5.8 g × 5 mL = 29 mL/hour

37 218.75 g
Step 1: Calculate what original strength of solution is
40 mL diluted to 500 mL to give 0.5% w/v solution
This is a dilution factor of 12.5 (500 ÷ 40) = 12.5
Diluted 12.5 times gives us a 0.5% w/v solution
Original concentration must be 12.5 times stronger than this
0.5 × 12.5 = 6.25% w/v
Step 2: Calculate how much potassium permanganate is needed to
give 3500 mL of a 6.25% w/v solution
6.25% w/v = 6.25 g in 100 mL
Multiply by 35 to give 3500 mL
6.25 × 35 = 218.75 g

38 4 days
Step 1: Calculate daily dose
Dose = 35 mg/kg
35 × 32 = 1120 mg daily
Step 2: Calculate how much 250 mg/5 mL suspension needed to give
1120 mg
250 mg ÷ 5 mL = 50 mg/mL
1120 mg ÷ 50 = 22.4 mL daily
Step 3: Calculate how many days 100 mL will cover
100 ÷ 22.4 = 4.46 days

39 18.75 mg
Step 1: Using table, determine BSA for a 12 year old
LS = 12 years old = BSA 1.25 m^2
Step 2: Calculate weekly dose
1.25 × 15 = 18.75 mg

40 2 g
Step 1: Calculate creatinine clearance
Creatinine clearance (mL/min) = $\frac{1.04\,(140-82)\times49}{150}$
= 19.70 mL/min
Step 2: Determine level of renal impairment
eGFR = 10–25 mL/min/1.73 m^2
Therefore need to adjust dose

Use half normal dose every 12 hours
Step 3: Apply dose adjustment
Unadjusted dose is 2 g every 8 hours = 2 g per dose
Therefore need to half the normal dose and administer every 12
hours
= 1 g BD maximum daily dose
= 2 g daily

SECTION D

1 9 mL

Tablets dose: 500 mg. Bioavailability is 75%. 75% of 500 is 375 mg (active bioavailable product)

The oral dose should achieve a bioavailable amount of 375 mg. Therefore, 375 mg is equivalent to 85%, so 100% is 441 mg. Suspension is available at 50 mg/mL. Dose is therefore 8.82 mL. Rounded up to 9 mL

2 2000 mL

Maximum volume of fluid/water she should receive = 30 mL/kg × 65 kg = 1950 mL

In practice you would hang a full bag of fluid, so this patient should receive 2000 mL maximum

Maximum amount of glucose she should receive is 100 g

5% glucose = 5 g in 100 mL = 100 g in 2000 mL

Therefore, she should be given no more than 2000 mL glucose 5% to ensure she does not become fluid overloaded

3 97 mg

BSA = $\sqrt{([\text{height (cm)} \times \text{weight (kg)}] \div 3600)}$

BSA = $\sqrt{([170 \times 80] \div 3600)} = 1.943650 \text{ m}^2$

Dose = 50 mg/m^2 × 1.943650 m^2 = 97.1825 mg. Rounded to nearest mg = 97 mg

4 1.2 mL

The SPC states: The loading dose should be administered in divided doses with approximately half the total dose given as the first dose and further fractions of the total dose given at intervals of 4–8 hours

Therefore, total LD = 600 microgram

First portion is 300 mcg

Vial is 250 mcg/mL

Total volume of digoxin needed = (1 ÷ 250) × 300 = 1.2 mL

5 7 mg

2 × brown = 2 × 1 mg = 2 mg

1 × pink = 1 × 5 mg = 5 mg

Total dose = 7 mg

6 22.75 mL/min
Candidates are expected to know the formula as it is commonly used in practice.
CrCl = (140 − age) × weight × F (F = 1.04 female, 1.23 male) ÷ serum creatinine
CrCl = (140 − 70) × 51 × 1.04 ÷ 162 = 22.75 mL/min

7 24 mmol
6 tablets per day × 4 mmol per tablet = 24 mmol

8 32 days
480 ÷ 15 = 32 doses
One dose a day, so 32 days

9 20 g
Use of alligation method can be implemented here

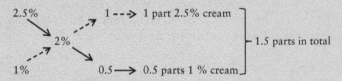

Need to make up 60 g so 60 g ÷ 1.5 parts = 40 g/part
Therefore, 40 g/part × 0.5 parts = 20 g 1% cream to be used

10 10 ampoules
Each ampoule has 200 mg/mL × 10 mL = 2000 mg per ampoule
Infusion 1: 150 mg × 55 = 8250 mg. This is 5 ampoules worth
Infusion 2: 50 mg × 55 = 2750 mg. This is 2 ampoules worth
Infusion 3: 100 mg × 55 = 5500 mg. This is 3 ampoules worth
Total ampoules needed: 5 + 2 + 3 = 10 ampoules

11 29.875 g
20 mg × 15 = 150 mg morphine
2 g base initially needed (to be displaced): 2 × 15 = 30 g
Displacement value is 1.6. Therefore 1.6 g of morphine will displace 1 g of base

Need 200 mg (0.2 g) of morphine. This will displace 0.125 g
Therefore total base needed = 30 − 0.125 g = 29.875 g

12 15 mL

Need 15 mmol calcium (Ca^{2+}), therefore need 15 mmol of calcium
chloride hydrate ($CaCl_2 \cdot 2H_2O$)

Convert from g/mol to mg/mmol, which is equivalent. Therefore you
have 147.01 mg/mmol

Utilise and rearrange molar equation: moles = mass ÷ molar mass
→ mass = moles × molar mass

Therefore mass of $CaCl_2 \cdot 2H_2O$ needed is 15 mmol × 147.01
mmol/mg = 2205.15 mg

14.7% = 14.7 g in 100 mL, therefore this is 147 mg/mL

2205.15 mg ÷ 147 mg/mL = 15.00 mL

13 6 mL

Patient is taking 120 mg total of background morphine

Minimum dose for breakthrough pain is 1/10th of the total daily
dose

Therefore: 120 mg ÷ 10 = 12 mg

10 mg ÷ 5 mL = 2 mg/mL

Dose is 6 mL

14 75 tablets

Draw a table to calculate the dose

Dose	No. days	No. 5 mg tabs per day	Total no. tabs
30 mg	5	6	30
25 mg	3	5	15
20 mg	3	4	12
15 mg	3	3	9
10 mg	3	2	6
5 mg	3	1	3
Total			75

15 225 g

Concentrations stay the same – only change is liquid paraffin made
up to 250 g

Draw up a table for ease:

Ingredient	Amount	For cream (250 g)
Calamine	4%	10 g
Zinc oxide	3%	7.5 g
Glycerol	1%	2.5 g
Macrogol	2%	5 g
Paraffin	Up to 250 g	X

Total liquid paraffin $= 250 - (10 + 7.5 + 2.5 + 5) = 225$ g

16 1820 mL
100 ml/kg for first 10 kg $= 1000$ mL
50 mL/kg for 11 – 20 kg $= 500$ mL
20 mL/kg for 21 – 36 kg $= 320$ mL
$1000 + 500 + 320 = 1820$ mL

17 4 suppositories
SmPC states:
Children under 3 months of age (60 mg suppositories)
One suppository (60 mg) is suitable for babies who develop a fever following immunisation at 2 months. Otherwise only use in babies aged less than 3 months on a doctor's advice.
Method of administration
These doses may be repeated up to a maximum of 4 times in 24 hours. The dose should not be repeated more frequently than every 4 hours. The recommended dose should not be exceeded.

18 5.8 micrograms/kg/min
500 mL at concentration of 0.05%
$0.05\% = 0.05$ g/100 mL
Therefore, there is 0.25 g/500 mL. This is equivalent to 250 mg/ 500 mL
The rate of infusion is 42 mL/hour
Therefore, to work out how many mg are being infused per hour is $250 \div 500 \times 42 = 21$ mg/hour
Now convert to micrograms/kg/min: 21 mg $= 21000$ microgram
The patient weighs 60 kg, so the infusion is $21000 \div 60 = 350$ micrograms/kg/hour
Need to work out per minute: $350 \div 60 = 5.83333$ micrograms/ kg/min

19 1.6 mL
200 mL × 20 = 4000 mL final solution
1 mg in 5 mL = X mg in 4000 mL
4000 ÷ 5 = 800
4000 mL will contain 800 mg
Therefore there is 800 mg in the original 200 mL
The stock of 50% w/v = 50 g/100 mL
50,000 mg in 100 mL = 500 mg/mL
800 mg = 1.6 mL concentrate needed

20 202 mg
Two batches of 400 plus 1% (404)
Total injections = 808 injections
Each injection = 1 mL
Therefore 808 mL required
250 mcg/mL → 250 × 808 = 202, 000 mcg needed
202, 000 mcg = 202 mg

21 130 mcg
S_{cr} (mg/100 mL) = (95 × 113.12) ÷ 10,000 = 1.07464 mg/100 mL
C_{cr} = (140 − 75) ÷ 1.07464 = 60.485371
% daily loss = 14 + (60.485371 ÷ 5) = 26.0970743
Maintenance dose = 500 × (26.0970743 ÷ 100) = 130.48537 mcg
Digoxin needed = 130.49 mcg
Rounded to the nearest whole number is 130 mcg

22 8 drops
60 mcg × 57 kg = 3420 mcg = 3.42 mg
= 3.42 mg/hr = 0.057 mg/min
150 mg/1000 ml = 0.057 mg/0.38 mL
20 drops = 1 mL, so in 0.38 mL = X drops
X = 7.6 drops = 8 drops

23 160 mL
1% of 40 mL (initial concentration and volume)
Final solution should be 0.2% in X mL
Can use C1V1 = C2V2
1% × 40 mL = 0.2% × V2
V2 = (1 × 40) ÷ 0.2

V2 = 200 mL
Started off with 40 mL so final answer = 200 − 40 = 160 mL

24 1.44% w/v
The SPC states: a dose of 40 mg/kg is needed
Therefore the dose for this patient = 18 × 40 = 720 mg
720 mg/50 mL = 1.44% w/v

25 1.6 QALYs
14 months = 1.166666 years
QALY best supportive care = (1.166666 × 0.5) = 0.5833333
37 months = 3.083333
QALY product = (3.083333 × 0.7) = 2.1583333
QALYs gained = 2.1583333 − 0.583333 = 1.575
Answer to 1 decimal place = 1.6
Please note that this question has been significantly simplified for ease. Normally we would look to adjust a lot more factors to ensure the populations to be analysed are as comparable as possible to reduce risk of bias and heterogeneity.

26 11.5%
Moles = Mass ÷ RMM
2 ÷ 23 × 1000 (to convert to mmol)
Total sodium allowed is: 86.9565 mmol per day
Patient is taking 2 × 5 mmol doses a day = 10 mmol
Percentage is (10 ÷ 86.9565) × 100 = 11.5%

27 250 mg
Vd for patient: 0.4 × 70 = 28 L
Required plasma level of 6.2 mg/L
28 × 6.2 = 173.6 (bioavailable product)
173.6 mg = 0.7 (bioavailable)
Therefore 173 ÷ 0.7 × 1 = 248 mg = oral dose (prior to absorption)
Rounded up to 250 mg

28 1 bottle
4 drops QDS = 16 drops per day × 7 days = 112 drops
20 drops per mL = 5.6 mL
= 1 bottle to be supplied

29 £2.10

Product	Cost	Cost per tablet
Esomeprazole 20 mg tablets (28 tablets)	£2.24	£0.08
Omeprazole 20 mg capsules (28 capsules)	£5.55	£0.1982
Amoxicillin 500 mg capsules (21 capsules)	£1.15	£0.0548
Clarithromycin 250 mg tablets (14 tablets)	£1.30	£0.0929
Metronidazole tablets (21 tablets)	£4.10	£0.1952

Regimen 1: omeprazole 20 mg BD, clarithromycin 250 mg BD and metronidazole 400 mg BD (7 days)
$(0.1982 \times 2 \times 7) + (0.0929 \times 2 \times 7) + (0.1952 \times 2 \times 7) = £6.8082$
Regimen 2: esomeprazole 20 mg OD, amoxicillin 1 g BD and clarithromycin 500 mg BD (7 days)
$(0.08 \times 7) + (0.0548 \times 2 \times 2 \times 7) + (0.0929 \times 2 \times 2 \times 7) = £4.6956$
Cost difference: £2.1126, rounded to nearest 10p = £2.10

30 1340 mg
The SPC states:

Dose modification of gemcitabine within a cycle for bladder cancer, NSCLC and pancreatic cancer, given in monotherapy or in combination with cisplatin

Absolute granulocyte count ($\times 10^6$/l)	Platelet count ($\times 10^6$/l)	Percentage of standard dose of Gemcitabine (%)
>1,000 and	>100,000	100
500–1,000 or	50,000–100,000	75
<500 or	<50,000	Omit dose*

*Treatment omitted will not be re-instated within a cycle before the absolute granulocyte count reaches at least 500 ($\times 10^6$/l) and the platelet count reaches 50,000 ($\times 10^6$/l).

Monotherapy
The recommended dose of gemcitabine is 1000 mg/m^2, given by 30-minute intravenous infusion. This should be repeated once weekly for 3 weeks, followed by a 1-week rest period. This 4-week cycle is then repeated. Dosage reduction with each cycle or within a cycle may be applied based upon the grade of toxicity experienced by the patient. This patient requires 75% of the standard dose.

ANSWERS

BSA for patient is 1.788854 m^2
Dose is $1000 \times 1.788854 \times 75\% = 1341.64$ mg. Rounded down to 1340 mg

31 343.75 L
22 000 ppm = 22 000 g in 1 000 000 mL
This is equivalent to 2.2 g per 100 mL. 250 L contains 5500 g
One batch has 110 bottles, each producing 25% w/v. 250 mL $\times$ 25% w/v $= 62.5$ g. $62.5 \times 110 = 6875$. Need to include 10% overage $= 7562.5$ g needed
Concentrated material: 250 L = 5500 g
Work out litres required for 7562.5 g: $7562.5 \div 5500 \times 250 = 343.75$ L

32 0.008% w/v
800 mg in 250 mL $\rightarrow$ diluted 1 in 40 = 10000 mL
Therefore, 800 mg in 10000 mL
800 mg in 10000 mL = 8 mg in 100 mL = 0.008% w/v

33 29 mcg/kg/hour
Oral dose: 30 mg BD = 60 mg/day
Parenteral dose will therefore be 30 mg/day
Dose will be $(30000 \text{ mcg} \div 43) \div 24 = 29.0697$ mcg/kg/hour

34 £410 pounds

Strength	*Biquelle* XL	Cost per tablet	*Mintreleq* XL	Cost per tablet
300 mg tablet (60 tablets)	£74.45	£1.240833	£49.99	£0.83316667
400 mg tablet (60 tablets)	£98.95	£1.649167	£64.99	£1.08316667

Dose	No. patients	Cost of *Biquelle* XL per day	Cost of *Mintreleq* XL per day
800 mg	120	£395.8	£259.96
600 mg	250	£620.4166667	£416.5833333
400 mg	130	£214.3916667	£140.8116667
Total cost		£1230.608333	£817.355

Difference per day = £1230.608333 – £817.355 = £413.2533333
Rounded to the nearest £10 = £410

35 £40

Strength	*Biquelle XL*	Cost per tablet
300 mg tablet (60 tablets)	£74.45	£1.240833
400 mg tablet (60 tablets)	£98.95	£1.649167

If 40% of high dose patients change

Dose	Current patient numbers	Current costings	Projected patient numbers	Projected costings
800 mg	120	£395.8	72	£237.48
600 mg	250	£620.4166667	298	£739.536667
400 mg	130	£214.3916667	130	£214.391667
Total		£1230.608333		£1191.40833

Total daily savings = £1230.608333 – £1191.40833 = £39.200003
Rounded to the nearest £10 = £39.20

Index